49 WAYS TO SEXUAL WELL-BEING

DR FRANCES CARTER

49 WAYS TO
SEXUAL
WELL-BEING

A practical guide for women

DR FRANCES CARTER

First published in Great Britain in 2015 by Step Beach Press Ltd Brighton

© Dr Frances Carter

The right of Dr Frances Carter to be identified as the author of the work has been asserted in accordance with the Copyright, Designs and Patents Act 1988.

A CIP catalogue record for this title is available from the British Library.

ISBN 978-1-908779-09-0

Picture credits: depositphotos.com

Series editor: Jan Alcoe

Typeset in Brighton, UK by Step Beach Press Ltd

Printed and bound by Spinnaker Print, Southampton

Step Beach Press Ltd, 28 Osborne Villas, Hove, East Sussex BN3 2RE

www.stepbeachpress.co.uk

49 Ways to Well-being Series

If you have selected this book, you may be looking for practical ways of improving your well-being. If you are a health and well-being practitioner or therapist, you may be helping your clients to improve theirs by encouraging them to practise some of the approaches it is based on. Well-being is a subjective state of 'feeling good' which has physical, mental, emotional and even spiritual dimensions. Because these dimensions overlap and interact, it is possible to improve well-being by making positive changes in any one. For example, taking up regular exercise (a focus on physical well-being) may improve concentration (mental well-being), happiness (emotional well-being) and sense of purpose (spiritual well-being). This series of well-being books is designed to provide a variety of routes to recovering, sustaining, protecting and enhancing well-being, depending on your interests and motivations. While some emphasise psychological techniques, others are based on physical movement, nutrition, journaling and many other approaches.

Each book in the series provides 49 practical ways to improving well-being, based on a particular therapeutic approach and written by an expert in that field. Based on tried and tested approaches from its field, each title offers the user a rich source of tools for well-being. Some of these can be used effectively for improving general resilience, others are especially helpful for particular problems or issues you may be dealing with, for example, recovering from illness, improving relaxation and sleep, or boosting motivation and self-confidence.

Enjoy dipping into any *49 Ways* book and selecting ones which catch your interest or help you to meet a need at a particular time. We have deliberately included many different ideas for practice, knowing that some will be more appropriate at different times, in different situations and with different individuals. You may find certain approaches so helpful or enjoyable that you build them into everyday living, as part of your own well-being strategy.

Having explored one book, you may be interested in using some of the other titles to add to your well-being 'toolbox', learning how to approach your well-being via a number of different therapeutic routes.

For more information about the series, including current and forthcoming titles, visit **www.stepbeachpress.com/well-being**

CONTENTS

FULFILLING SELF

CONFIDENCE

PLAY FANTASY FU

FUN SEXUALITY LIFE

SENSUALITY CHANG

SELF PLEASURE CURIO

INDIVIDUALITY

COMMUNICATE EXPLORAT

GSPOT FLIRTIN

RELAXATION PUBLIC EROT

AGEING YOGA TO

BODIES MOVEMENT YOU

MASTURBATION ORGA

PERSONA STEREOT

DISABILITY PAIN PRIVA

FEMALE EMPOWERME

ACKNOWLEDGEMENTS

Thank you to Dr Martin Edwards GP, writer and columnist, and to Emma Cole, yoga instructor and blogger for their expert contributions to this book.

Introduction

This practical yet informal guide aims to bring you an increased awareness of your sexual potential, to help you increase your sense of yourself as a sexual being. It suggests that it is by acknowledging the significance of our sexuality to our sense of who we are as individuals, that we can increase both our well-being and our being in the world. *49 Ways to Sexual Well-being* prioritises an awareness of individual, innate sexuality as a part of living well with oneself and others: lovers, friends and strangers. In a tone at once light-hearted and practical, the author suggests a wide range of strategies which may be used to support sexual exploration, whether the reader is single or in a relationship.

For a long time women have experienced challenges in pursuing any exploration of their autonomous sexuality; much media material focuses on how to be more sexually appealing to men or how to re-ignite a sexually flagging relationship. This book works on the premise that sexuality pervades every aspect of our daily lives, whether we are walking the dog or buying the Sunday papers. While the guide is written primarily with women in mind, it hopes to provide food for thought and sexual practice for everyone, regardless of gender, age or sexual preferences. My hope and intention is that dipping into this book will help you to ignite your sense of sexual self-confidence, guide you in finding new avenues of sexual self-pleasuring, and give you permission to uncover and enjoy the abundance of sexual frisson to be found in everyday experience!

In preparing to write, I talked to a number of women about some of the themes I aimed to cover, and in fact, their kind participation informed both the content and the structure of the book. My rather informal research ranged widely – I talked to women about a range of issues, from how to maintain a sexual self as you grow older, and how to imbue your home with sensual pleasure, to the controversial topic of female ejaculation. I have included short quotes from these conversations in many of the 49 Ways and I am indebted to all the women who spoke to me for both their insight and their tolerance of my foraging into the most intimate areas of their lives. It is in no small part thanks to their contribution that this book takes such a very broad perspective regarding female sexuality.

Overall, *49 Ways to Sexual Well-being* aims to acknowledge the utter centrality of sexuality to all our lives, whatever our age, background, gender or sexual persuasion. This is not a book about re-igniting your sex life, this is a book about re-igniting your sense of self!

How to use this book

Rather than being overwhelmingly problem orientated, a common focus of many sex guides, this book focusses on positive suggestions for embracing your sexuality. Throughout the book there will be passages to get you thinking about yourself and your relationship to sexuality. There are light hearted and hopefully useful exercises aimed at helping you to see yourself in an increasingly sexual light, as well as personal views, insights and experiences from the women I have talked to in the course of writing this book.

While I suggest you start with the first Way – which is designed to start you considering your sexuality as a personal attribute rather than something to be viewed in relation to others – essentially this is a book to dip into. Each themed chapter is separated into five Ways, most of which include a 'Try this' activity as an invitation to put some of the ideas in practice.

1 2 3 4 5 6 7 8
9 10 11 12 13 14
15 16 17 18 19
20 21 22 23 24
25 26 27 28 29
30 31 32 33 34
35 36 37 38 39
40 41 42 43 44
45 46 47 48 49

Chapter 1

THE SEXUAL YOU

This chapter focuses on preparing to acknowledge your own sexuality through experiencing yourself as an autonomous being in the world.

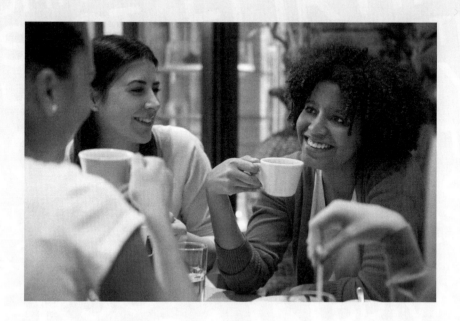

1 Sous la buffet?: Engaging with yourself and the world as a sexual being

'Zazou est disparu sous la buffet'. This is a line probably misremembered from my old French school text book; the story of Zazou who was perpetually lost beneath the sideboard. These days whenever something I once had is lost, I automatically associate it with the tiny French boy lurking under an obsolete piece of furniture. Where has my sexuality gone? It is underneath the sideboard.

It is easy for us to lose touch with our sexuality. Female sexuality is complex, not simply on an individual level but also in terms of the 'bigger picture'. We view female sexuality through various lenses, some of which make it difficult to understand just what feminine sexuality might look like or to see our own sexuality in a way that looks familiar, understandable or comfortable to us. In the media, overtly sexual women are often portrayed as highly self-confident, even predatory or 'man-eating'. On the other hand, the sexual woman may be depicted as needy or emotionally unstable – often a combination of the two. This style of presenting the sexual woman may be off-putting or alienating to us. Bombarded by media imagery, we tend to associate the highly sexual woman with youth, beauty and the frenetic consumption of things which promise to provide us with those very qualities we lack. Overwhelmingly, we conflate being sexual with being found sexually attractive by others.

- Think of five women who are thought of as 'sexual' – they could be celebrities, politicians or people you know. Deduct five points if you include Helen Mirren (just joking).

- Have a look at your list. Think about whether these women are attractive to others or simply appear comfortable in their own skin.

- Now subtract the candidates who are on the list because they are described as beautiful or sexy.

- Who's left? What do these women have in common? Do you like them? If so, what is it that you like about them? Can you describe what it is it about them that makes you think of them as sexual women?

This is not a book designed to make you more attractive to others, although there is every chance that with a new found sense of self, you may become so! This is a book that hopes to keep you company on a journey of sexual self-discovery. There are many personal reasons why we might lose sight of ourselves as the sexual beings we undoubtedly are. We may be in a long term relationship which has gone a bit stale, or not in a relationship at all. For various reasons, we may lack the everyday confirmation of an active sex life and some-body who wants to make love to us. We may be so busy that we have lost this side of ourselves somewhere between Sainsbury's and the staff car park. Our children might have stolen it from us; there is nothing like the burgeoning sexuality of teenagers to make you wonder what happened to your own! Perhaps we never felt that sexual a being in the first place and we are simply wondering what it feels like to be one – must we suddenly turn into a pouting, unfeasibly pneumatic blonde bombshell? Perhaps the most obvious reason that we may lose sight of this side of ourselves is ageing. It is a truism, particularly for women, that we live in a culture dominated by the notion of youth. But take some time to look around you and you will see many older women who are bright, engaged, attractive well into their seventies and eighties. These are the women we must celebrate. Look at old interview footage of the now departed Lauren Bacall in her 70s, sitting ramrod straight, still alluring, her caustic, pithy wit intact while she defied every stereotype of the older woman. You will find many examples of your own.

Over the course of this book we will start to explore the idea of ourselves as sexual beings. We will discard the notion that validation from others is the objective and the barometer of our sexuality. You and I will be re-discovering our sexuality together, exploring ways of expressing ourselves as sexual beings, not as sexual clichés. Our focus will be on being, not doing – although there may be some doing, it will be doing for ourselves rather than for others.

2 First steps to feeling good about your sexuality

Everyday life can sap your sense of self, never mind your sense of your sexual self. We are often caught up in the world of work, our domestic responsibilities, concerns about our children and, as we age ourselves, our parents. We do things to try to please others and we judge ourselves by whether we are managing to keep everybody else happy. Overwhelmingly, we find that we identify ourselves in relation to other people as mother, partner, colleague, daughter, friend, employer or employee. Of course, all these roles and relationships entail intense pleasures as well as a whole raft of responsibilities and obligations, but it is difficult to maintain a sense of ourselves as sexual beings in the face of all the other things we are!

In order to regain this understanding of who we are as individuals, to re-kindle our capacity to take action independent of other's needs, and vitally to rediscover ourselves as sexual beings, it is vital to recall sometimes that we are also separate, self-determining human beings. By this I mean that while a view of ourselves as autonomous agents can be eroded by the pressures on us to be this or that to him or her, we can find ourselves again in small ways and in unexpected places.

Try doing something this week, however small, just for yourself. Don't yawn, swear at me or shut the book! Being told to do something for yourself *is* a cliché of women's magazines and self-help manuals, but we are repeatedly told to do this because it is undoubtedly something that, as women, we sometimes forget to do. I believe that you cannot begin to experience your own sexual self when you are fully occupied being something or someone to somebody else, that before you are sexually stimulating to others, you must be sexually alive to yourself. For this reason, it is vital to engage with the world, just sometimes, as *yourself*, without apology, without regret and without commitments. A short cut to achieving this is to put yourself in a position where the people around you know nothing about you and to allow yourself to luxuriate in that feeling. Find time to be, not simply *by* yourself, but somewhere you can actively put aside commitments and obligations. Try to make these small moments a part of your week. Be careful about what you choose. Go swimming because you enjoy the feel of the water on your skin, don't tell yourself that you are going because your body needs toning up. Try shopping with no particular aim or motive, allow yourself to pick something you fancy on the spur of the moment. Make sure you don't go looking for appropriate work clothes, an outfit for a wedding or even something to make you look appealing to your partner – this should be shopping at its most selfish and luxuriant!

- Sitting in a café with a cappuccino is a good time to be with yourself by yourself. Not too demanding in terms of time spent away from other demands, it's a chance to be still, to notice the world around you, to interact with others in a way that is purely superficial... and nobody can tell themselves that they are sitting in a café for the sake of their inner thighs!

- Try not to think about what you need to do that day, don't use the time to make a 'to do' list. For these few moments simply be there, anonymous, another face in the crowd. Notice other people, allow yourself to be curious about them and realise that they may be curious about you. Make up stories about who they are in your head and realise that somebody may be doing the same about you.

- Now! Remember your list of sexual women and pick one. Imagine yourself as her. Try to emulate her self-confidence for a moment as you sit in the café. How would she sit, arrange her legs, order a second cappuccino? Imagine yourself as her, surveying the room and being surveyed in turn. We are having a bit of fun here but visualisation is a very useful tool and we will be using it again.

WAY 3

Hoop earrings are clearly the way forward

I hope you managed to do something for yourself, however small and seemingly insignificant that might be, but something that in a very small way began the process of reminding you of your own *'beingness'* in the world. Do try to hold onto this idea and prioritise spending some time in every week doing something by yourself, something that allows you a personal satisfaction and enjoyment, this is a first step to re-engaging with yourself as a sexual presence.

Inevitably we conform to the behaviour that is expected of us at every life stage. It took me years to admit that I do not enjoy music festivals and I remember in my early 20s sitting, shivering slightly with cold and boredom, trying to arrange my face in a suitably rapt expression but actually wishing it was all over and I could go home to bed, preferably with a hot water bottle and a cup of tea. Now I have reached some small level of middle aged security in who I am and what my preferences are, I can happily admit that I really like 70s disco and while I can completely understand the historical and cultural importance of rock music, I'm happiest blasting out a bit of Chaka Khan and shaking a bit of booty.

What's more, I know that I can feel more myself when I am not in a relationship, not necessarily happier, but somehow my sense of who I am gets slightly eroded in trying to live up to the inevitable expectations and preferences of somebody else, not to mention the domesticity that eventually and inevitably seems to dominate most relationships. Perhaps it is simply that outside a relationship one is able to be more open to possibilities, more prepared to take a risk and put in the effort required to try something new. A few beers and a box set on the sofa with your partner can seem very attractive on a drizzly Friday night. To prevent your sexual identity getting lost in the morass of 'everydayness' that is our day to day experience of relationships, work, parenthood and so on, it is important to do small things that allow you to remember who you are as an individual; after all, if you have a partner, it is this individuality, those insignificant quirks that originally attracted them to you and you to them!

- One short cut to this is to draw on your past. Is there a period that you look back on with affection and some pride, a time when you felt brave and attractive and revelled in revealing yourself to others, a time when you felt other people not only responded to you positively but responded to you in a way that made you feel you were funny, interesting and attractive? This time might be a moment, a day, a summer or a decade.

- Now that you have identified this time, a time when your confidence in yourself was, maybe not soaring or exultant, but secure – is there something in your memories of yourself that you identify with that period, event or moment in your life? Was this a time in your life when you wore a lot of vintage clothing, painted your toe nails blue or wore a specific brand of trainers? Was this a time you associate with a particular type of music or even a food? Of course, if you had a wonderful summer in Cyprus when you were 19, I am not suggesting heading straight out to Ayia Napa, but I do want you to do some small thing that ignites not only the memories, but the feelings you had about yourself at that time. For example, what about that toe ring?

- If this isn't working for you, try another tack. Is there some small thing you have always wanted to wear but have never felt confident enough to wear? For example, I have always wanted to wear hoop earrings, but have habitually told myself that I don't feel I have the right face shape, the right look and in any case, I'm too old. But perhaps I could just wear them anyway!

So perhaps you have now gone down to Accessorise to get yourself a toe ring, bought some feta cheese, made a Greek salad, put on some very loud house music and rediscovered those positive feelings about yourself that you once had. Whatever you have managed to do, don't expect anything much more than a fleeting feeling of nostalgia or a brief sense of pleasure in something remembered. But bear in mind, this is just one of 49 Ways and 49 tiny steps to igniting your sexual self and to help you get Zazou out from sous la buffet.

Lost between the stacks

'I looked at a sex manual with a friend when I was a teenager and we laughed like drains, but kept looking and tried to remember to put it back in exactly the same way.'
Jodie 37, Graphic designer

We have begun by thinking about your sense of self and what psychologists have sometimes called, 'self-actualisation', that is, a state in which one feels one reaches a level of true potential, in this context sexual potential. To this end I hope you have accessed a memory or started to revitalise a sensation of the person you are, beyond your work, home or relationships. Perhaps this sensation is invested in some sort of talisman, an object, smell, sound or taste which re-ignites those confident and optimistic feelings you had about yourself at that time. For me, let's say it is the hoop earrings that embody or materialise this state of mind. Presently, we must start to bring sensuality in, to build on that fragile sense of autonomy we are creating by making gentle links between the autonomous, self-actualised person – and the sensual or sexual person.

You may wonder why I am putting so much emphasis on the idea of the person as separate, independent, autonomous – sex after all, is largely represented as something one does with somebody else. However, I believe strongly that sex is not only an act engaged in by one, two (or more!) individuals, but it is also a part of the way in which we engage with our world and with our daily life within that world.

If you search in a book shop for the section which deals with sexuality, it often forms a part of the shelving labelled 'relationships', 'self-help' or 'health and well-being'. Well, where else would it go? However, these labels make several assumptions which form part of our '*taken for granted*' understanding of female sexuality. Firstly, the idea that our sexuality serves a relationship with somebody else – usually assumed to be a masculine else – we *work on it* in order to improve our relationship with our partner. The second label, self-help, reinforces this notion, we must *work on* our sexuality, it is a project – like building a shed! Clearly, we don't have it quite right and it can be improved if we follow expert guidelines, pay close attention to the easy-to-follow diagrams and extend its life by assiduously applying wood preserver every year. Lastly, if sexuality is part of health it must also be part of its corollary, illness. Therefore, it is either healthy or it is sick and if it is ailing, then yet again, we must strive to make it better, to make it fit a universal model of 'healthy' sex. This approach simply makes me feel exhausted.

'Sex manuals – when found in someone else's house, read avidly!'
Lucinda 37, Personal assistant

'Sex manuals are for people without any imagination. I find the explicitness off putting.'
Eliza 48, Masseur

We come to sex, and we leave it as individuals; it is not an act in which two people merge and become one, for each participant experiences the sex they are having differently. Nor is it a process which attempts to achieve a perfect union or flawless performance arrived at through consensus. Since everyone and every one of their partners will have different expectations, inclinations and preferences it is difficult to become 'better at it'. After all, what leaves one partner swooning in sweaty and contented satisfaction may leave another partner wondering how quickly they can get up and make a cup of tea.

Our sexuality and the way in which we practise sex, is part of our individual personhood. It is whom we choose to be and what we are as the result of the totality of our experiences. By this I mean that our sexuality and how we enact sex is inevitably a response to our previous experiences of sex, our broad understanding of what sex is all about, what it encompasses and what place it takes in our lives. Mediated representations of sexuality and societal pressures to be sexual in certain prescribed ways unavoidably shape both our likes and dislikes and own performance of sex. Ultimately, we bring our distinct sexuality to the act of sex with ourselves and with others, for sex is not a cooking contest in which we are all striving to create the ultimate fondant fancy.

So where else in Waterstones could the sex manual go? How about: 'science fiction and fantasy', 'history' or my own choice, 'autobiography'? Where would you put your own sexual story?

WAY 5 Doing sexuality

We have established that sexuality is about being and pleasing yourself, not simply about providing a pleasurable experience for another person (although a sexual experience *may* sometimes be primarily about giving pleasure to somebody else). We have introduced the idea that your sexuality is a part of your identity and as such it is an encounter with your independent, autonomous self rather than yourself in relation to others. So far we have prioritised how you *think* about yourself in relation to your own sexuality. Here we focus instead on physical sensation and the body. These suggestions are simply a bit of fun – pick and mix them as you fancy and start gathering some ideas of your own! Begin by exploring the sensation of different textures next to your skin. For example, you might try not wearing anything to bed. If you usually wear pyjamas, a nightie or an old t-shirt, try sleeping in nothing at all. If it's not the middle of summer take a hot water bottle to bed or turn on your electric blanket. Luxuriate in clean sheets and indulge in the sensation of them next to your skin. Try contrasting textures, wear something very soft or something heavy like thick wool or light silk with nothing underneath. You don't have to go out like that, just experience the sensation for a short while. My mother used to have a fur coat and I vividly remember trying it on with nothing underneath, then I turned it inside out...!

My most profound experience in relation to fabric and texture was washing a pair of leather gloves. A friend had some gorgeous white kid gloves which had got rather dirty. She found that you could buy glove shampoo and taking a glove each, we washed them in the sink, rubbing our hands together in the suds. After a few moments we were both giggling and ooh and aaahing. Neither of us has ever forgotten it! We don't all have a handy pair of white kid gloves but you could start gathering sensual objects to keep in a box under the bed. This can be just a shoe box but you may add to this later (see Way 18) and might want to think about finding something more secure, particularly if there are other people living in the house with you! For now, think about gathering textures that feel good against your skin: velvet, fur or even rubber.

As well as physical sensation we can make use of the most powerful of our senses: smell. Massage oil or body lotion is an obvious route to awakening and enlivening your sensual self on two levels. Smell is considered to trigger memory more effectively than any other sense, and combining this with the sensation of gently stroking and rubbing your own skin can be a powerful sensual experience. Try not to allow yourself to make judgements about your body as you do this. There may be a part of your body you don't like, but tell yourself that by nourishing your skin you are looking after your body just as you look after it by eating well and exercising. Self-care is an important way of re-connecting with your sensual self. So do your best to block those habitual negative thoughts from your conscious mind. Another way to harness our olfactory senses is to wear something that belongs to somebody else, a friend or a lover; you will be subliminally conscious of their personal scent. Try wearing somebody's t-shirt because you love or admire them. You may even find that you briefly take on aspects of their persona, your best friend's vivacious manner or your partner's capable way of dealing with problems.

'When I first got interested in sex it was the Lynx affect. I really like armpit smell. If you're attracted to someone you've smelt them already.'
Jodie 37, Graphic designer

Lastly, try playing with the power of taste. If you have a partner, try taking it in turns to blindfold each other, then the seeing partner may feed the other a variety of different foods, one by one, and ask her to guess what they are. Try to find foods that not only taste different but feel different in the mouth, for example, a banana, a piece of tinned asparagus, jelly. This is something to have fun with but there must be a high level of trust between the two participants as it can be surprising how vulnerable one feels when blindfolded.

Play music and dance to it in the privacy of your own home. In the Further Information, Reading and Resources section there is a suggested playlist but of course this is an individual preference: play something that makes *you* want to dance and play it loudly. If there is a window through which a neighbour might see you, turn the light off or better still leave it on and enjoy the idea of being watched – even just for one song. We don't dance enough as a culture and it's something we shouldn't save for weddings or the occasional Friday night out. Move your whole body and aim to get breathless from the exertion; the sensation of uninhibited rhythmic movement is a significant means by with we can get in touch with a dormant or temporarily sluggish sensuality!

References

Alcoe, J., Gajewski, E. (2013) *49 Ways to Think Yourself Well*, Brighton: Step Beach Press.

Wilson-Kovacs, D. (2009) 'Some texts do it better: Women, sexually explicit texts and the everyday', in *Mainstreaming Sex: The Sexualisation of Western Culture*, London: I. B. Taurus.

1 2 3 4 5 **6 7 8**
9 10 11 12 13 14
15 16 17 18 19
20 21 22 23 24
25 26 27 28 29
30 31 32 33 34
35 36 37 38 39
40 41 42 43 44
45 46 47 48 49

Chapter 2

EVERYDAY SEXUALITY

You don't have to take dancing and burlesque classes, but you can!
This chapter is focused both on those with and without a partner.
Having begun to think about your sexual self in relation to the world,
here we start to explore relating to others in a sensual context.

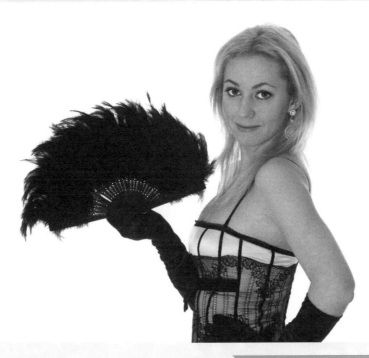

WAY 6 — Overcoming the challenges to a fulfilling sex life without a partner

Being without a long term partner need not mean that you cannot *be* and fully enjoy your sexual self. Indeed many women feel at their most alive and sensual when not in a relationship. The freedom of being single can mean a woman is open to all kinds of daily opportunities to explore or live out desires, preferences and experiences that may enhance her sense of herself in sensual relationship to the world. After all, relationships can become mundane and domestically driven, and it is more than possible to lose your sense of self in the demands of catering to the needs of another. Therefore, living for and pleasing yourself may offer women a less circuitous route to actualising their sexuality in everyday life.

For some of us, however, it is true that staying in touch with ourselves as sexual and sensual beings when not in a sexual relationship can be a challenge. It can be difficult to access a belief in one's sexual desirability without the confirmation that a sexual relationship, at its best, can provide. But please note here my caveat, 'at its best': many long term relationships do not provide this sort of on-going ratification of our sexual attractiveness. As a single woman you can have a world of stimulation and sensual validation at your disposal with nobody to reign you in, be envious or jealous, or provide you with an unwelcome and possibly questionable interpretation of your actions. Furthermore, I hope that if you have read this far, you will be familiar with my proposition that feeling sexual is not dependent on being desired, in fact, *feeling* sexual is more likely to *lead* to being desired!

Some of the ideas outlined in this section about feeling sexually alive without a partner are suggestions designed to encourage you to engage with others in a way that brings your sexual *beingness* to the fore; others are simply suggestions of ways in which to put you physically in touch with your surroundings and with others.

Singing is sexy! We have already mentioned music, but singing is an activity which facilitates an immersion in your own physicality. What's more, it can be uplifting, stimulating and arousing. In order to produce a perfect sound, you must work on your breath, your posture, your tonal affinity with those around you, your ability to project your voice – the same attributes that you must use to flirt in fact!

As well as singing for your own enjoyment – for example, I tend to sing in the car – consider more social singing in a choir or at a workshop. The common goal to produce a wonderful (or not so wonderful!) sound can be an immense aphrodisiac, at the very least binding you with others in a shared physical endeavour. While singing alone enlivens the senses, perhaps, ironically, singing with others can be a powerful route to finding one's sense of self – a self in relation to others. This might even give you the opportunity to try out your flirting techniques – see Way 7.

'I find singing in a group really exciting, particularly when you're performing in public. There's something about the edginess of trying to find your way, blending with your own section, listening to the other parts, which is totally absorbing. And then there can be moments of real emotion and even ecstasy when you hear a particular harmony.'
Tasha 51, Local government worker

As well as singing, keep up the dancing! There are all sorts of dance classes for which you do not need a partner. For example, I have tried Lindy Hop and although it is a partnered dance, most classes will move students from partner to partner so going alone is not a bar to a great evening's dancing. Recently I was reminded how much I would like to learn to do flamenco, a supremely sexual dance – a solitary display of a woman's sensual power and allure made more potent by her physical relationship to the music.

7 Flirting for fun only

Flirting is a good way to re-ignite an inherent sense of sexual and sensual power. It is often said that flirting is a muscle that must be exercised. Inevitably there are many, many reasons why we stop exerting this flirting muscle, or perhaps we have never located it in ourselves and so never start to flex it. We may be prevented from flirting by a lack of confidence, a sense of ourselves as growing older, or a belief that it is no longer appropriate for us to flirt. Flirting may stop being a part of our lives as we get ever more caught up in dailyness. As we have already seen (see Way 2), we may think of ourselves primarily as parents or carers, rather than as attractive or sexual beings. We may feel that it is a style of behaviour that is not for us, that denotes a certain type of overtly 'up for it' woman. However, I think that the main reason we stop, or perhaps don't even start flirting is because of a myriad of misconceptions and misplaced beliefs about what flirting is, what it means, what it says about us and what it might lead to.

We have talked a little bit about stereotyping the 'sexy' woman. To many of us she is in her 20s, has long blonde hair, peachy but heavily made up skin, and a bee stung pout glistening with lip gloss. Sexy woman wears tight denim shorts or skirt and a t-shirt which is at least a couple of sizes too small. She always wears high heels and her default facial expression is along the lines of 'come hither'! Sexy woman hangs out in bars, scanning the room to see who is available. The raison d'être of sexy woman is to attract men; she appears vacuous and empty-headed but underlying this, she has poor self-esteem and her sense of herself is only validated when she has secured the interest of some equally empty-headed male!

'Other women don't like women who flirt all the time: short skirt, blonde hair, Barbara Windsor, loose, a predator, the giggly type.'
Jodie 37, Graphic Designer

Jodie's outdated image of the sexually predatory woman is one defined by the tabloid press and none of it is what we are about here – if any of this even bears the slightest relation to what you think of as a sexual women and flirtatious behaviour then recap from Way 1!

I prefer to think of flirting as being beguiling, charming, compelling, an allure achieved largely via the strategy of surprise. A successful flirt is rarely explicit and never crass. A successful flirt creates a world inhabited, momentarily perhaps, by two people.

'Flirting is teasing!'
Lucinda 37, Personal assistant

A successful flirt fashions a brief alliance which declares 'there is us and then there is the rest of the world'. Flirting has very little to do with age or beauty and is only occasionally a precursor to sex. It does however, require a certain confidence and being comfortable in one's own skin.

Of course that ability to exhibit flirtatious charm has many and varied components, but I would characterise it as a capacity to make others feel good, interesting, funny and appreciated but with that additional and vital component. Many people are kind, empathic and good listeners but do not use their undoubtedly excellent qualities in a flirting offensive. They lack the ability, confidence or desire to create that extra frisson of surprise – the major constituent of successful flirting behaviour!

- Spend a few minutes picturing somebody flirting. It might be a person you know or an imagined person. How do they look? What are they wearing? What is their expression and what are they saying and doing? What is their tone of voice like and how are they standing or sitting? Try to make this image as colourful, detailed and large as possible.

- Once you can see this person and visualise their flirting behaviour, try to encapsulate your image in a few key words – between five and ten. It doesn't matter how disjointed or meaningless these words seem initially.

- Now have a good look at the words you have used to describe your flirting image. What do they reveal about your perception of flirting? Are there aspects of your visualisation which seem positive and fun, or conversely, are there aspects of it which raise difficulties for you?

Successful flirting needs a light touch and 'stereotyping' may get in the way of finding a way of flirting that works for you. A woman I spoke to when researching this book was advised at a flirting workshop to picture a man's crotch while talking to him – this seems to me akin to taking a sledge hammer to crack a ripe peach (although she reported it working for her!) Being aware of how you visualise flirting and the flirt is the first step to allowing yourself to find a comfortable, light-hearted and, most of all, enjoyable way to dally with the man or woman at the dry cleaners.

WAY 8

The fearless flirt: how to do it

When I have to go to an interview or another situation in which I do not feel entirely comfortable, I often use the technique of pretending to be somebody else. This strategy of modelling the behaviour of another can be very successful when you start out or return to flirting after a flirting break. Who can you think of who has the ability to flirt? How do they operate? What is it about their flirting behaviour which is so appealing?

'It's complimenting other people, sometimes people read a little more into it though. You just have talk to them basically, don't you?'
Jodie 37, Graphic designer

What do I mean by *surprise*? In the context of flirting what I am suggesting is the introduction of an element which is very slightly outside of expected, conventional behaviour for that social situation. I will give you an example. Ellie is naturally bossy and outspoken. While this can be a negative attribute in some contexts, for her it is highly effective when she is in the mood to flirt. When in a social setting our usual mode of behaviour will involve listening attentively, showing empathy and indicating agreement. Try to recall when you were last at a party: didn't you find yourself standing with your head slightly to one side, nodding effusively and laughing in all the right places? Picture Ellie in the same situation, slightly strident and engagingly severe, she bucks the social trend by unexpectedly telling somebody that they are quite wrong, by giving them a ticking off, by telling them just what they should be doing or would be far better off having done! Of course tone is vital here, Ellie will do this with a light, almost ironically school ma'am-ish touch which often catches her quarry off guard. It is this 'catching off guard' which I would suggest is the aim of the fearless flirt. Aim for the unexpected!

'Whenever I order a whiskey on the rocks, I always get a reaction. It differentiates me from the rest of the girls in the pack with their glasses of white wine!'
Theresa 27, Post grad student

Give yourself a chance to flirt. Every encounter can be flirtatious – no need to distinguish between the middle-aged man in the dry cleaners and the attractive and available friend of your best friend's husband. I don't believe that you can't do it, but If you *think* you don't know how to flirt, here are some guidelines, some serious and some less so!

• Lower your chin ever so slightly so that you are looking up at the person you are speaking to.

• Lower your voice and speak a tiny bit more slowly than usual.

• Develop stillness, since stillness and reticence is more successfully flirtatious than agitation.

• Use small, slowly emerging smiles.

• Make very slightly more eye contact that would be usual for that type or context of social encounter. Then look away.

• Touch your face more than normal, particularly a gesture which allows you to play insouciantly with your lips – perhaps against the palm or fingers of one hand.

• The most important two flirting techniques are to look interested in what the other person says and to find an excuse to touch their arm, lapel or some other non-sexual, innocuous part of the body.

Compliment someone, then when they are lulled into a sense of security, de-stabilise them by gentle teasing or saying something challenging.

WAY 9 A world of sexy things: the significance of good knickers

We live in a world of 'things', and we are encouraged to locate our sense of self, and identity in our consumption of those things. For example, a particular type of moisturiser promises to give us back our youth, a high heeled shoe will make us look sexy, owning the right sort of toaster will show that we have the right sort of taste. Our identities are bound up with what we buy and what others can see that we own.

Sexuality is often expressed in terms of things. We are sexy if we wear a tight-fitting dress or a snake-print blouse artlessly unbuttoned at the neck; we are sensual if we wear a scent advertised by a particular celebrity currently promoting her latest role which contains several risqué sex scenes with the latest hot acting talent. Sexuality is conflated with objects that have little to do with sex in our everyday worlds, such as cars, coffee and cat food. Advertisers and marketing companies know that we are vulnerable to the notion that we can acquire or consume sexuality by purchasing a particular washing powder, and undoubtedly this is partly because we are not secure in our own innate sexual identities.

Rather than struggle with the inevitable irritation we might feel when faced with a negotiation between our sense of self and the world of objects, let's bow to the inevitable! We live in a material world so let's talk clothes!

Try this

List the colours that you tend to wear most often and then try asking yourself these questions:

- What do you think those colours say about you and what associations do these particular colours have for you?

- Now add to the list the colours you feel most evoke sexuality, and say why.

- What colours make you feel most like yourself and most sexually alive, which make you feel dowdy or unappealing? Which ones do you usually find yourself wearing?

- Go back to the visualisation exercise we did in Way 2. Recall the women you identified then as being 'sexual'.

- Don't limit yourself to celebrities: are there women you know who you feel are good with clothes or have a personal 'look' you admire? How would you describe their 'image', what shapes do they wear and what colours? Do they use accessories or is their look very pared down? What could you adopt and adapt for yourself?

The most sensual women are those who look as if they are comfortable in their own skin; that means feeling relaxed in what you are wearing. If you don't find heels comfortable, don't wear them, pain and discomfort is attractive to no one worth bothering with.

Personally I get annoyed by advice that purports to suggest what is appropriate for women to wear at particular ages. You know the sort of thing – what to wear in your 20s,30s, 40s, 50s and so on. By the time you get to 40 all the models are in floaty scarves, mid length skirts and short layered haircuts. So for goodness sake break the mould!

It is undoubtedly a truism touted by every woman's magazine but nobody feels sexy or sensual in baggy, greying underwear. Most women probably have special underwear that stays in a drawer for the occasion that never arises. Worn once or twice it is a silent reproach to those of us who think, 'No it's too uncomfortable, I can't be bothered'. But this is the wrong way to think about underwear. Don't think about wearing it for somebody else, stop envisaging pulling on your scratchy red thong only for your partner to wince slightly at your sagging buttocks. Go back to that old adage, 'What if you were run over by a bus?' What you need is underwear to be run over in, something not overtly sexy perhaps but underwear that you wouldn't mind being seen in, something comfortable but well-fitting and most of all – matching. The effect of matching underwear is something akin to magic. It instantly makes you feel sophisticated, attractive and well prepared. Try a simple t-shirt style in beige, brown or peach – French women rarely wear coloured underwear! Sophisticated colours such as black, navy blue and camel tend to make me feel more alluring; I struggle to feel sexy in brown but feel free to disagree about its delights!

WAY 10 Your home is a boudoir

So far we have focused on ways to feel sexy which involve some level of working on the self. Just for fun let's think for a moment about how to make your environment one which sets the scene for a new, more sexually alive you.

'Clean sheets and a good bed. Get rid of the kids and the dog and draw the curtains.'

Eliza 48, Masseuse

Here I need to make an admission: while the rest of the house is not too bad, nothing could be less sexy than my bedroom currently and I feel utterly fraudulent in making any suggestions to anybody else. However, I did say at the outset that we are on a journey together and this Way is one where I will most certainly be acting on my own advice! So join me as I strip the bed and sort through my drawers!

Lighting is obviously a significant factor in terms of creating a sensual environment. Overhead lighting should be banned for all but the most practical of tasks. Clearly candles not only hide a bit of dust and cracks in the walls, but are flattering to both you and your home. Don't, however, reserve candles for special evenings. I once worked with a woman who, when I knew her, was in her 80s and lived alone. She made a point of lighting candles every night for her own pleasure. The memory of this woman has stayed with me for many reasons, but one of them is her admirable resolution to enjoy this small, sensual pleasure every day.

Think about texture: in a world when so many luxuries are out of reach, good quality bedding is something that may be worth investing in. A really good pillow or two as well as high thread count sheets will add hugely to the experience of reading an erotic novel at bedtime!

I have a hunch that a bed works less well as a site of sensual pleasure if there are innumerable and sundry objects hidden under it. Try and keep the 'things under the bed' to a minimum.

'Having clutter everywhere is not sensual, it's anxiety-making. And open the windows so you can smell the season.'

Eliza 48, Masseuse

Importantly, try to keep technology out of the bedroom. The bedroom should be a place of relaxation and sensual comfort, it should not be a place to catch up on your email. Having said that, we will make *some* exceptions to that rule (see the appendix to Way 15 for online sources of erotic pleasure which you may want to take *into* the bedroom).

- Set yourself one small task, the accomplishment of which will make your home into something more of a sensual haven – even if temporarily! For example, smell can be an aspect of the domestic setting which may radically influence not only the way you and others experience your home, but can alter the ambiance of the home, according to the effect you are trying to create. There is no need to spend a fortune on scented candles and please, please never use plug in air fresheners. Flowers can be used to scent individual rooms or try a few drops of vanilla essence on a metal tray heated gently in the oven for 10 minutes or so.

'The scent of vanilla is very evocative because I associate it with a particular loved one. Bacon sandwiches in the morning, homely food smells all do it for me.'
Jodie 37, Graphic designer

The slightly serious message behind this Way is that creating a more sexual you means not only focusing on sexuality itself but a re-thinking of all aspects of your life – and that includes the environment in which you live. A home which meets your needs for sensual experimentation is one which need not be perfect in any sense, but allows for the possibility of some small sensory delights, such as a vase of daffodils, a soft blanket, the smell of something mildly exotic in the oven – things that can contribute to your sensory pleasure and ultimately impact on your sexual well-being.

1 2 3 4 5 6 7 8
9 10 **11 12 13 14**
15 16 17 18 19
20 21 22 23 24
25 26 27 28 29
30 31 32 33 34
35 36 37 38 39
40 41 42 43 44
45 46 47 48 49

Chapter 3

FANTASY AND FRISSON

This chapter looks at the part that fantasy plays in women's sexual experience. Here we focus on dispelling those stereotypes of fantasy or arousal that frame or limit our understanding of female sexuality. We start by exorcising some of the myths around what it means to be a sexual woman; then we look at the role fantasy plays in our everyday lives, moving into the nitty gritty of self-pleasure, and lastly, a few thoughts on women's relationship with erotica and pornography.

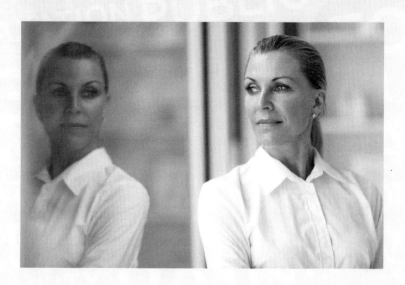

When you get right down to it!

While men may joke with their friends about 'pulling the pudding', female masturbation remains something of a taboo subject. Partly this is because, until comparatively recently, masturbation by both genders was considered not only to be immoral and indicate weakness of character, but moreover, to be the cause of all sorts of ills and diseases. Even today there are traces of some of these anxieties and misconceptions. Masturbation is still sometimes talked of as an activity of the lonely and un-partnered, spoiling one for 'real' sex, or even de-sensitizing the male and female genitals. Even today there are traces of some of these anxieties and misconceptions. Masturbation is still sometimes talked of as an activity of the lonely and un-partnered, to spoil one for 'real' sex, even to de-sensitize the male and female genitals. In discussion of masturbation one may still encounter the misleading notion that the ease of achieving solitary pleasure can threaten women's potential enjoyment of partnered sex.

'I try to keep it as something to do when I don't have a partner so that I enjoy it more with them; it's too easy to do it yourself. You want your partner to get skilled at it, if you keep doing it yourself you'll never get a good one with them. I think your orgasms get a bit weak and feeble if you masturbate too much.'
Jodie 37, Graphic designer

It is extremely difficult to determine what proportion of women masturbate; clearly so much guilt and embarrassment surrounds the subject that accurate reporting is unlikely. For some of us self-stimulation is loaded with so much that is challenging that we don't allow ourselves to enjoy touching our own bodies at all.

'Nowadays I don't think about masturbation, it doesn't occur to me as an option. I think I've always felt guilty, goodness knows where that came from. I've always had lots of guilt issues.'
Lucinda 37, Personal assistant

Whether we do it to relax, to get to sleep, because we are frustrated, bored or have a headache, most of us masturbate or have done at some stage in our lives. What seems to be apparent is that frequency of masturbation is not dependent on whether or not women are in a relationship. Whether we masturbate, or how often, is likely to have much more to do with our cultural beliefs about female sexuality, perhaps our religious beliefs and, of course, our sex drives. It might be that an early formative experience has shaped our view of self-pleasure, for example, we may have been brought up in an atmosphere of sexual inhibition. What is vitally important is to remove and discredit any negative associations that may colour how we think about masturbation. I suggest that if we do not know how to bring ourselves to orgasm, it is hard to explain to anyone else how to pleasure us sexually.

Try this

- We live in a culture which finds female sexual self-expression of any kind problematic; furthermore some women find the idea of self-stimulation a difficult one for myriad reasons. If that is the case forget about masturbation or orgasm for now and focus on simply allowing your body to luxuriate in pleasurable sensations.

- This could simply mean clean sheets and a hot water bottle (one of my ultimate pleasures!) or it could mean a hot bath with expensive bath oil and an evening on the sofa in cashmere bed socks.

- Giving ourselves time and permission to indulge our bodies in whatever way feels pleasurable and that allows us to feel relaxed in our own skin *is* important and something we should all make time for. At times (or for some women) this sort of relaxed indulgence of the senses may be pleasure enough in itself!

A hot bath or hot water bottle *may* make you feel that you want to take this further, but I'm guessing that some other form of stimulation will be required if you want to excite and satisfy yourself sexually. Fantasy is a vital element in achieving arousal, and while many women can access fantasy easily by replaying a memory or imagining a stimulating scenario, others may need some sort of external stimulation and there are suggestions for this in Way 14. The next Ways focus on exploring our own fantasies.

WAY 12 Making it our own

It is an often repeated truism (nevertheless absolutely spot on) that sex begins in the mind – in other words, in fantasy. Whether or not we have a partner, fantasy is a natural part of everyone's sexual repertoire. A life mired in the routine, the commonplace or domestic, in a way of being which rejects or excludes fantasy, will mean that inevitably we cease to think of ourselves in sexual terms. However, fantasy can be an alarming word, particularly 'perhaps' for women. It can conjure up ideas of the forbidden or the perverted. Alternatively, someone who fantasises may be thought to be out of touch with reality; at the very least a propensity to fantasise might suggest to some that one is unhappy or dissatisfied with the reality of life.

I suggest that we need to make friends with the notion of fantasy. An active fantasy life can inject new life or excitement into an existing relationship, but may also prompt new ways of thinking about ourselves and ourselves in relation to others. Sexual fantasy can perhaps be broken down into categories: fantasies about the self; fantasy about another or others; fantasy concerning place or context; and finally, fantasy about the act itself – whatever that might be. Stereotypically, most people utilise fantasy for self-stimulation in the seclusion and privacy of their own homes. But, of course, sometimes the frisson of excitement may be embodied in the unexpected or 'jarring' combination of various elements: let your fantasy life enliven a dull Friday afternoon in Sainsbury's, for example!

- Download a mildly erotic audio book onto a portable device, but rather than listening in private, take it to a café and enjoy the frisson of enjoying something mildly titillating in a public space.

WAY 13 Women and fantasy

There are many myths and orthodoxies around women and sexual fantasy.

For example, there is a pervasive notion that women have less interest in visual stimulation than men. While men are supposedly reliably aroused by visual representation of the sex act, we are told that women watching erotica are focused on the *context* of a sexual encounter; the relationship between the protagonists, the back story, the curtains! Women are often said to need a romantic plot, to require tasteful scenarios played out on nice quality bed linen before they can feel aroused.

While this may be true enough for some, this way of talking about female sexuality can mean that those of us who don't fit that fantasy stereotype are left feeling that we are outside the feminine norm, or even guilty about the nature of our fantasy life. Thus for the very many women who do find looking at pornographic or erotic material sexually arousing, with or without attendant flouncy window treatments, these stereotypes may be problematic, leaving women questioning the legitimacy of their preferences. In fact, there is also much quoted research which suggests that women are just as aroused by explicit visual stimulation as men, but for whatever reason, are unable to admit to the stimulating effects of viewing sex on a screen. If this research has any validity, then the disconnection between what *actually* arouses many women and what they *think* arouses them is worryingly subject to societal pressures around what women are *supposed or allowed* to find sexy.

Given all the myth making around female sexuality, I think it is vital to start thinking about what stimulates and excites you as an individual. Of course it is hugely difficult, if not impossible, to put to one side all those things which are either supposed to interest and excite you, or on the other hand, are supposed not to. However, if we are to reach an understanding and acceptance of our own predilections, (or at the very least a rapprochement!) we must allow ourselves to investigate what those predilections might be. We must allow our imaginations free reign and attempt to silence that internal (or sadly external) voice which strives to fence in our fantasy worlds.

Give yourself ten minutes somewhere quiet and secluded:

- Replay in your head a scene from a film, a television series or a book that you have found sexy or arousing in the past. Give the scene as much visual detail as you can, allow yourself to completely enter into it. You won't remember it in minute detail, but let your own imagination fill in the bits that you have forgotten. See the environment where the scene took place, visualise the lighting, the textures and colours of the surroundings, the physical position of the people. Replay the action, the words the people say and the sounds they make (make it up if you can't remember, you will have the gist of it). Attempt to empathise with how the characters are feeling – first one character and then another. Allow yourself to wallow. Give yourself at least five minutes.

- Then take a pen and paper: I want you to unpack in single words or brief phrases what it was that you found sexy about your scene. Start with individual visual elements, then perhaps get more abstract or emotive, highlight particular details that you enjoyed.

- I am hoping that having done this once (or perhaps twice with another of your favourite scenes) you will find that the elements *you* find exciting have very little to do with any sort of stereotypical imagery. I am willing to bet that there are few words or images in there that bring to mind a 24-year-old pneumatic blonde pouting and lowering her eyelids at a deeply moustachioed man!

In fantasy you have the licence to explore whatever takes *your* fancy. In fantasy you have complete control over what happens, as well as the freedom to enjoy being anybody you wish and to enjoy anybody or any body, you wish. In fantasy you never have to explain your preferences or deal with any consequences. I'm not suggesting that you should walk around in a sheer white chemise in a constant state of falling off one of your snowy white shoulders but, hopefully, I am prompting you to begin to access what *you* find exciting, sexually stimulating or arousing.

WAY 14 A fantasy source guide!

Having asked you to start investigating what it is you find arousing, I'm going to contradict myself and offer a few ideas of my own, as well as the thoughts of women I have interviewed for the purposes of writing this book.

'Literature can be very arousing. It's a private experience, evocative isn't it? But it can't be in your face.'
Lucinda 37, Personal assistant

Erotica and sex guides

Nancy Friday talks about women's erotic lives in what, in the early 1970s, were groundbreaking terms. Today her work remains a mainstay of feminist writing about female sexuality and female sexual fantasy. Her books are discussions about and collections of, real women's fantasies described in their own words, for example:

- *My Secret Garden: Women's Sexual Fantasies* published in 1968
- *Forbidden Flowers: More Women's Sexual Fantasies* published in 1994
- *Women on Top: How Real Life Has Changed Women's Sexual Fantasies* published in 1991

'*Women on Top* has been on my bedside table for 20 years or more. I read it when I can't get to sleep or whenever I feel that sexual itch. It never fails to make me feel aroused when I need it to, but over the years it's also been a comforting read; just to find that women fantasise about so many things, some of them a bit strange, makes me feel I'm in good company.'
Celia 46, Teacher

The Good Vibrations Guide to Sex by Cathy Winks and Anne Semans published by Cleis Press. From the pioneering San Francisco sex shop, this erotic manual has advice for lovers of all persuasions. It is strong on practical 'how to' style advice as well as what to buy – good for browsing and entertainingly written.

The Lovers' Guide Interactive. The Ultimate Guide To Sex DVD by Robert Page, produced in collaboration with the relationship charity Relate. Topics include sex toys and sustaining sexual desire in a long term relationship.

A few films variously suggested to me as arousing (in the broadest sense!)

Don't Look Now 1973, directed by Nicolas Roeg, includes one of the most famous sex scenes of film history; it is also one of my favourite films!

Out of Sight 1998, an engaging American crime film directed by Steven Soderbergh and based on the novel of the same name by Elmore Leonard.

In The Cut 2003, an Australian-American mystery and erotic thriller written and directed by Jane Campion and featuring a surprisingly sexy performance from Meg Ryan.

I Am Love 2009, an Italian film directed by Luca Guadagnino and featuring a relationship between wealthy Tilda Swinton and a much younger man.

Secretary 2002, directed by Steven Shainberg and (very sympathetically) featuring a mildly Bondage Discipline Sado Masochism (BDSM) relationship. Highly recommended if you haven't seen it, a film to inspire discussion if nothing else.

Almost anything by Spanish film maker Pedro Almadovar.

My Beautiful Launderette 1985, a groundbreaking and affecting British film dealing with a same sex and inter-racial relationship.

'I watched *My Beautiful Launderette* in the '80s when it was a ground-breaking film on various fronts. But also, maybe surprisingly, I remember finding it deeply arousing. Perhaps it was the tenderness of the relationship, or the difficulties and prejudices the characters were dealing with, I don't really remember but i do remember it was really hot!'

Celia 46, Teacher

Damage 1992, a British-French film directed by Louis Malle and featuring a transgressive relationship in which Jeremy Irons has an affair with his son's partner, played by Juliet Binoche.

Body Heat is a 1981 American neo film noir written and directed by Lawrence Kasdan. It was inspired by *Double Indemnity* and stars William Hurt and Kathleen Turner.

'*Body Heat* is set in the southern states and I remember this as a very sultry film. There was a lot of sweaty tanned male body and Katherine Turner in flimsy white dresses, it was all about what was going to happen – so your imagination can run wild. Like 9½ weeks but so much better!'

Françoise 51, Print shop owner

Blue is the Warmest Colour 2013, directed by Abellatif Kechiche, is a romantic and highly sensual coming of age drama about two young girls.

See the Further Information, Reading and Resources section, Way 15, for a list of female erotic film makers.

Some literary (or not very!) erotica for every taste

Eleven Minutes by Paulo Coelho (2003) is based on the experiences of a young Brazilian prostitute.

Secret Life of Catherine M by Catherine Millet (2001) is the 'true' story of a French art historian and her sexual encounters.

Venus in Furs by Leopold von Sacher-Masoch (1870) deals with themes around sado masochism and female dominism.

Possession by AS Byatt (1990) follows two modern-day academics as they research the love life of two famous fictional poets.

Story of O by Anne Descios (1954) is the story of a sex slave. Notorious and controversial, over recent years it has been re-appropriated as a classic text about sex.

Fanny Hill by John Cleland (1748) is a bawdy and very explicit romp, illuminating in terms of the sexual mores of 18th century England but also a real turn on!

Scruples by Judith Krantz (1992) is a classic 'transformation' novel. Billy evolves from overweight poor relation to thin stylish rich girl. Of its time but a bit of fun.

Anything by Edmond White, one of our foremost contemporary novelists and also a writer whose work is explicit in its depiction of gay sexuality.

Delta of Venus by Anais Nin (1978) comprising interlinked short stories set in the world of the Paris *demi monde*. Originally written in the 1940s, it is a staple of feminist literature on sexuality.

Tropic of Cancer by Henry Miller (1934) is a novel in which a highly sexed man explores the sexual possibilities on offer in Paris.

Couples by John Updike (1968). One of our best contemporary writers on sex and relationships.

Lost Girls by Alan Moore (2009) is a graphic novel that explicitly imagines the sexual adventures of three fictional characters, Alice (in Wonderland), Dorothy (from *The Wizard of Oz*) and Wendy (from *Peter Pan*).

Black Lace has been publishing erotic fiction, by women and for women, since 1993. I have never read one but many women do!

The final Way of this chapter focuses on what is on offer on the web.

15 Sex in cyber space

The women's movement has had a troubled relationship with pornography which is still very much in evidence today. During the late 1970s and early 1980s, feminist debate was polarised between anti-porn groups and those in the movement who took a sex-positive position. The view that much pornography degrades and objectifies women is highly prevalent and largely unarguable. Of course, I recognise that pornography, even female orientated pornography, is a highly controversial topic and something that for many women remains a no-go area – both for personal and political reasons.

'I've got really strict rules about porn because I think it's exploitation. It's not real, it's removed, it's on a screen, that would make me a voyeur. I don't like the perceived predatory aspect of the internet, I don't feel it's sexy.'
Eliza 48, Masseuse

While internet porn is currently blamed for innumerable societal ills, pornography tends to be discussed as if it is *all the same* or all of it equally offensive, while in truth pornography as a genre is as enormously varied as film or literature. For those women and their partners who are seeking sexual pleasure, stimulation or information, there are a large number of women-friendly websites and sources of material that seek to show women as active participants in, and initiators of, pleasure rather than simply as objects of masculine desire.

'Porn can be educational in some ways, it can give you ideas, because it's not necessarily really sordid – it depends what you choose to watch. Some people can be totally in love.'
Jodie 37, Graphic designer

There has been some research that points out that the anonymity of online sex has provided a new forum that allows women to explore the variety of their sexual desires, freely and in private. The internet can provide a useful platform for women to try out any number of fantasies without committing to actually living them out in their everyday lives. Online you can be whoever you want to be and dip a toe in any number of sexual streams, rivers or lakes. The internet can introduce you to new pleasures, to sources of information, even to new friends, but of course while there *are* excellent websites dealing with sexual matters, and very many which are designed particularly with women in mind, it is possible to become immured in sexualities that are not to your tastes. Furthermore, the web is at once a private and a public space and it is vital to exercise a level of caution and common sense when communicating online.

The Further Information, Reading and Resources section to this Way offers a preliminary guide to some useful online resources at the time of writing. This will, I hope, show the cautious that there is much fun and interest to be had online, as well many blogs, review sites and platforms for discussion around sexual issues which may or may not be useful, instructive or enlightening. Many of these are American rather than British in origin, and it is unavoidable that they vary in terms of quality and interest, as well as representing a very small selection of the websites on offer.

While some or all of the resources listed may not be for you, I hope that readers will be encouraged by the evidence that many women are attempting to re-frame and re-make erotica in the interests of women. I hope, too, that there is a discussion to be had around women, sexuality and the internet, and that the topic will not be dismissed out of hand – in effect, excluding women from all that new sexual representations may have to offer by lumping everything into one basket marked '*Pornography, it's for men*'.

See the Further Information, Reading and Resources section for this chapter for suggestions on some interesting and useful discussion and review websites as well as a list of female erotic filmmakers.

1 2 3 4 5 6 7 8
9 10 11 12 13 14
15 **16 17 18 19**
20 21 22 23 24
25 26 27 28 29
30 31 32 33 34
35 36 37 38 39
40 41 42 43 44
45 46 47 48 49

Chapter 4

SHOPPING FOR SEX

'In a climate where women are encouraged to be actively sexual, yet
have inherited a tradition which provides them with little idea of how
to manifest this, the pole, like lingerie and sex toys, may also "stand in"
for women's sexuality and give them the means of articulating it.'

Feona Attwood (2009, p178)

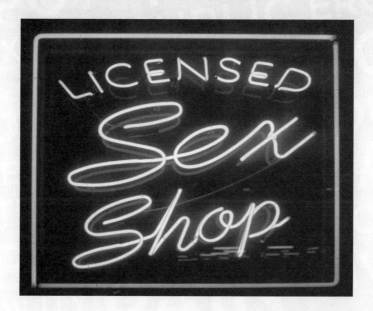

WAY 16 The stereotype of sex shopping: don't let it get in the way of a fun day out!

This chapter is going to look at sex shopping, a contradiction you may say, for in Way 1 we tried to dispel the myth of sexuality as a commodity, something to be bought in the flock wallpapered and luxuriously lit environs of an exclusive underwear boutique or in the shiny, bland whiteness of the cosmetics hall of a department store. However, here I am going to advocate sex shopping as an adventure: the actual purchase is not entirely the point!

The sex shop has undoubtedly still got an image problem. It is stereotypically conceived as somewhere exclusively for men, as sleazy, uncomfortable and embodying a style of sexuality perceived as hostile to women. Moreover, the term 'sex toy', a phrase usually used in connection with women-focused products, may be viewed as condescending and infantilising. I have such concerns myself, however I use it here in the absence of an alternative term that doesn't feel overly clinical.

Many women's first real encounter with a sex shop in the UK is via Ann Summers, which may be seen as offering an alternative to the blackened windows and nameless façade of the traditional sex shop. Ann Summers is highly visible on every high street, its window displays feature slightly raunchy underwear and its product range includes items with names such as Hustler Thrill Ride and Jiggle Wand. While Ann Summers has undoubtedly done much to break down the stigma of sex shopping for many women, it is not everybody's cup of tea. Its flippant, jokey and sometimes tacky style, evokes a raucous hen party approach to female sexuality, which may be just as off-putting for some as the Private Shop located on the fringes of most town centres.

The stereotypical male sex shop is usually licensed. Briefly, a licensed shop will sell hardcore pornographic material, such as R18 DVDs, along with 'toys' and other items. Some shops specialise in particular types of product, fetish wear or sado masochistic (S&M) products, for example. Gay sex shops also tend to be licensed and will sell a range of sexual paraphernalia alongside male lingerie. Licenses are supplied by local authorities and licensing criteria vary from area to area, but there will always be restrictions on what can be seen from the street or from an open doorway. If you are curious to visit a hardcore sex shop, it is my experience that gay shops are open and welcoming to women, as are the specialist shops which tend to be run by people knowledgeable and enthusiastic about their particular area of interest. A shop which is not licensed may sell softcore DVDs, books, magazines and sex toys, but the proportion of sexualised goods to the total stock must be lower, leading them to stock lingerie, bath products and massage oils in place of blow-up dolls.

Read on before you say, 'None of this is for me'. In many cities, sex or erotic shops are springing up which are unlicensed, and which cater to the sexual needs of women in a way which is inclusive, sensitive, unthreatening and fun. The early pioneers in terms of sexual retailing for women were Eve's Garden, which opened in New York in 1974 and, and famously, Good Vibrations, founded in 1977 in San Francisco. Both aimed to provide a sex-positive and female-centric counterpoint to the male orientated 'adult book' stores. Good Vibrations, in particular, supplied sex information and education and sold erotica and books about sexual health and pleasure. It sold sexualised items in open, friendly and light filled stores, forging the way for shops such as Sh!, arguably London's first women friendly sex shop, which opened in Hoxton in 1992. Like many of the shops which have followed these early pioneers, Sh! is open and friendly, you will be offered a cup of tea while you browse and the staff are knowledgeable and highly approachable. Many female-centric sex shops also operate a policy of forbidding men to enter the shop, unless they are accompanied by a woman (as the quotation from Celia shows) – a strategy which goes a long way to assist women in feeling comfortable and relaxed when sex shopping.

Every shop I have visited (and I've been to a lot!) will let you test the balance of the spanking paddles, taste the fruit flavoured lubricant and have a giggle at the wildly gyrating and passionately pulsating sex toys. More importantly, all these shops have customers from 18 to 80, and in none of them will you be made to feel in any way judged or uncomfortable. I have interviewed customers of a range of women orientated sex shops and all of them highlighted the mix of delicacy and straightforwardness, helpfulness and knowledge of the staff working in them.

'Well, to begin with it's in a very pretty part of town, it's a nice place that I enjoy going to, there's a nice little coffee house nearby and it's not in a district where you feel you have to duck in quickly in case anybody sees you. You feel fine to just walk straight in and then come out with a nice pink carrier bag with something lovely in it just for you!'
Francoise 51, Print shop owner

See the Further Information, Reading and Resources section for a list of women-friendly sex or erotic shops that you might try visiting, either alone or as part of a day out with a friend.

WAY 17

Make it social! Sex shopping with a friend

I hope the previous section began to dispel the stereotype of sex shops for those of you who haven't experienced the new breed of women's erotic emporium! I'm sure you are saying 'But most people sex shop online', and we will discuss that in a minute. Here I want to make the case for sex shopping as a social activity, and while of course you *can* shop online with a friend, there is no substitute for actually picking up a nipple pasty and wondering out loud together how to make it twirl!

'Because I went with my friend it was absolutely fine, we were chatting as we went in and we tried out things together and had a laugh. It just felt like we were going into any other shop really – but probably more fun!'
Celia 46, Teacher

Make sex shopping part of a fun day out with a friend, have a coffee or two, rummage in your favourite clothes shops and then pop along to the women's sex shop! (There is a list of suggestions at the end of this section). If you are at all nervous at the prospect, having a friend with you will instantly make you feel more comfortable. If you have a particular friend who you know is a sex shop aficionado, ask her to take you. Alternatively, share a new experience with another sex shop novice. Daring each other to try out something new can be great fun and the inevitable slightly embarrassed giggling is far more fun with two!

Sex shopping with a friend is an excellent way to stimulate what may turn out to be a seminal conversation. One woman I spoke to said that a friendship had been profoundly deepened by the experience of sex shopping together. Over a day's shopping and the purchase of a vibrator these two women had mended old fences and forged a new and lasting bond! This shopping trip was clearly a significant moment in their relationship, in purchasing something so intimate they had revealed aspects of themselves which may not have emerged in a day to day context. After all a mutual trip round Sainsbury's is unlikely to unearth hidden depths and secret lives – but it may!

However light-hearted the experience (and it should be!), inevitably you will end up sharing something of your feelings, experiences, preferences and prejudices about your own sexuality. Sex conversations are not only hugely fascinating in a prurient sense but an enormous source of pleasure, reassurance, fun and stimulation.

'Sex shopping is great if you're going for the experience of a giggly girls night out when you might want to try on things and just generally have a fun night out. But that's different to if you're going to buy something which you're going to use and is going to be quite pleasurable that hopefully you're going to be quite intimate with. You might want to go by yourself then.'
Tasha 51, Local government worker

Being a bit belligerent I've left shopping with a partner until last. A visit to a sex shop is often prescribed to couples as a way of spicing up their love life. I don't mean to downplay the value of this, but I'm determined that this should be a book about you. Having said that, going to a sex shop can be a way to add a sense of play to an already buoyant sex life with a partner. However, if your sex life is currently strained I would not recommend it. Go sex shopping when you are up for a bit of fun, happy to be experimental and prepared to play Star Wars with lots of sex toys with silly names. A shopping trip when one or both of you are stony faced and feeling dutiful is not likely to rejuvenate anything – in that situation concentrate on rejuvenating *you* for the moment and go with a good friend.

There is much fun to be had in sharing a new experience with another sex shop novice. Daring each other to try out something new can be great fun and the inevitably slightly embarrassed giggling while you work out how to twirl a nipple tassel or change the vibration and rotation speed of a wildly gyrating sex toy, is far more fun with two!

WAY 18

Beginner's guide to the tools of the trade

We have been discussing sex shopping because my own research shows that the *process* of sex shopping, walking into a shop, sampling the products, chatting about the experience, and so on, can in itself help a woman feel that sexual fulfilment is in her own hands – both literally and figuratively. However, the same research suggests that you don't actually have to buy anything! We are encouraged to feel, not least by the sex industry, that consumption is the route to all pleasure, but sexually speaking, you don't need to buy a single thing to achieve sexual stimulation, empowerment or fulfilment. Nonetheless, if you feel you would like to experience the additional stimulation potentially provided by owning your own tool then this Way is for you!

What will 'hit the spot' and where is the spot anyway? Buying a sex toy for the first time can be a somewhat daunting experience. Just like the confusion I feel when confronted by a myriad slightly different kinds of fabric softener, the tentative sex toy consumer may be put off by the enormous range of toys on offer. There may be confusion too about what these different types of paraphernalia actually do and who they are for, for example, do I really need a butt plug? Add to this the possible awkwardness, or even embarrassment, of shopping for something as intimate as haemorrhoid cream but with potentially more comedy value. This chapter is designed to dispel some of the mystery around sex toys but also to help you to identify what sort of toy might be right for you.

Look at the questions opposite. Hopefully by answering them you are starting to get a little nearer to identifying what *you* need from a sex toy. The next Way will tell you more about what is available.

Before buying a sex toy of any sort, think about what your sexual needs are. The following questions may help to guide you in the direction of, if not sexual nirvana, a bit of sexy fun!

- Do you want a toy for your solitary use or do you want something to use with a partner. Do somebody else's needs and fantasies need to be taken into consideration or can you please yourself?

- When masturbating do you focus exclusively on your clitoral area or do you feel the urge to have something inside you?

- Do you like to focus on one area at a time, or would the idea of vaginal and clitoral stimulation in tandem rock your particular boat?

- Do you like your clitoris touched firmly or is it so sensitive that you can only bear the lightest touch?

- Does the G spot feature in your masturbatory repertoire? (See Way 29 for more on the G spot.)

- What sort of textures might you prefer – something cold and hard or something warmer and softer? Many vibrators are now made of silicone; the advantages of this material are that it is soft and lifelike, it warms quickly to body temperature, is hypoallergenic and can be washed easily using soap and water. However, other materials feature in sex toy design. Dildos particularly are available in silicone, glass, wood, embedded with Swarovski crystals, double ended or ready to strap on.

- Is your bedroom in the east wing or do you live in a studio flat – in other words does the toy need to be as quiet as the tomb or can it make a satisfying buzz?

- Are you somebody who likes a crescendo and so may want to ramp it up as you near to a peak of excitement? In that case you may want a range of speeds.

WAY 19 All kinds of toys

There are, of course, all sorts of sex toys designed to meet the sensual needs of all women and, inevitably, to create sexual needs women didn't realise they had in the first place! However, the toys that most women will have encountered, either in conversation or in actuality, are dildos and vibrators. These terms are often used interchangeably, but a dildo and a vibrator are not the same thing. A dildo is not powered and therefore doesn't vibrate. Usually it resembles a penis, however abstractly; it has a shaft which is used for penetration of the vagina or anus. A dildo can either be used with the hand or as part of a harness (a strap-on); they can also be double ended for shared use.

Most women's first sex toy is a vibrator. A vibrator can be used alone for masturbation as well as with, or on, a partner. Vibrators come in many shapes and sizes but in essence they can be roughly penis shaped and designed for insertion in the vagina, or not penis shaped at all and designed to stimulate the clitoris or other strategic areas. They can be highly technical or simply switch on and off, but a vibrator 'does what is says on the tin' as it were – it pulses or vibrates. In addition many are now designed to stimulate two or more areas at once – the vagina, the G spot and the clitoris. The main types on offer are:

- **Rabbits**. There are any number of rabbit themed vibrators, including Thruster Rabbit and Thriller Rabbit. All are named after the original Rampant Rabbit which featured on *Sex and the City*. These will always feature a vibrating shaft for insertion into the vagina and two vibrating or moving 'bunny ears' which stimulate the clitoris at the same time.

- **Clitoral vibrators** are not necessarily even remotely penis shaped and certainly not all of them have bunny ears, although you will find a lot of ducks. Manufacturers such as *Lelo* and *Fun Factory* produce sex toys which bear little or no relation to the male member. These are primarily designed for clitoral stimulation and are a good starter sex toy for many women.

- **G spot vibrators** tend to be slightly curved at the tip to reach the G spot, while some also feature a clitoral stimulator. Some women find the G spot responds to pressure or firm swirling motions for which a specially designed vibrator may come in handy. (See Way 29 for more on the G spot.)

- **Finger vibrators** are tiny and have something in common with those novelty pencil rubbers, a party bag favourite, although of course these vibrate. They are designed to be placed on the end of a finger for solo play or discrete play with a partner. I have seen a Japanese brand featuring a range of anthropomorphic creatures designed to appeal to the enthusiastic sex toy collector.

• **Bullet shaped vibrators** are again discrete sex toys designed for the briefcase and handbag. Often deceptively powerful they offer clitoral stimulation in a discrete and non-threatening miniature package.

A last word on vibration. Vibrators come in a huge array of not only styles and designs but prices. Like anything else at the upper end of the range you are paying for the name and the status attached to it. Some are designed by well-known designers such as Tom Dixon and Phillipe Starck and many resemble sculptural objects. If aesthetics are an important part of your road to pleasure, then you may want to indulge in an upmarket designer vibrator. However, I suggest a starter vibrator should cost between £20 to £50. I cannot stress enough that if you want to buy a vibrator for the first time, or even fancy a new brand of technologically enhanced pleasure, go and see it and try it out first (this is certainly the time to try a visit to the new breed of women's erotic shops). You will need to hear how loud it is, feel the strength of the vibration and assess which functions are vital to you for experiencing pleasure. Once you have found something that works for you, by all means, buy online if that is more convenient. At the exploratory stage you will need to touch it, see it and hear it!.

See Further Information, Reading and Resources to this chapter for a list of woman-friendly sex shops in the UK.

References

Sex and the City, Season 1, Ep 9, *The Turtle and the Hare*, Aug 2, 1998.

WAY 20 That's (adult) entertainment!

'Burlesque – actually the idea of them is much better than the reality, mostly I think they are pretty tame and not at all erotic – more saucy postcard. It's quite nice seeing women being confident about their bodies and out there with their sexuality but some of them can be too much about male fantasy for me.'
Gabriella 45, Dental technician

This Way introduces some other ideas for exploring female sexuality, loosely under the banner of 'entertainment'. What all these things have in common is the idea of female empowerment. Today the term 'empowerment' embodies a range of meanings and images around the idea of women taking charge of every aspect of their own lives – from arguing for a stronger women's voice in politics, to the woman who is actively seeking out her own sexual pleasures. However, there is an argument that this idea has been cynically taken up as a marketing tool and devalued through overuse, that everything from a chocolate bar to the purchase of a new handbag has come to signal female empowerment. While I feel there is much truth in the idea that we are not emancipated by shopping, all of the things I talk about here have an investment in the idea of women being confident and comfortable with themselves as *actively* sexual, rather than as sexual objects.

All the women-centric sex shops I have researched have what we might call a 'sex-positive agenda', that is the belief that women should have access to not just sexualised goods, but sexual pleasure itself. Many such shops have excellent websites which, as well as selling products online, offer a range of information, help and advice on all aspects of sexual pleasure for those both with and without a partner. Some provide an online forum for women to share experiences and information or via which to ask questions of the sales teams, who have expertise well beyond the usual sales person when it comes to all things sex toy related.

In addition, some women's sex shops have an even wider remit and run classes, book readings and seminars on sexual matters. These are likely to be for women only and I have recently seen topics advertised at a well-known London store, such as beginner's bedroom bondage, strap-ons and pegging (prostate stimulation). My experience is that these classes are friendly, light hearted and informal events and a good opportunity not only to have an amusing night out with like-minded women, but enlightening and inspiring.

Pole dancing is a hugely contentious topic. While it undoubtedly conjures up the image of scantily dressed women gyrating around a pole for the delectation of hoards of slack-jawed men, it does have another and rather different incarnation. There are pole exercise classes springing up everywhere that operate a women only policy and profess to offer a safe, 'empowering' and highly effective exercise regime to women of all ages. This kind of appropriation – taking something with connotations around the objectification of women and re-making it in the interests of women – will always cause some to shudder. However, it is clear that for many women it is not only enormous fun, but a very bonding and self-affirming experience (particularly in terms of body image).

Lastly, a word about stripping and burlesque. What we think of today as the burlesque show has its roots in America around the 1860s to the 1940s. A kind of bawdy variety show that took place in clubs, music halls and theatres, it featured highly stylised female striptease. Since the 1990s, there has been a 'revival' of interest in the burlesque show, and where once it was rather 'fringe', it has become increasingly mainstream and commercialised. However, the idea persists in some quarters that burlesque is not just a sort of dressed up strip show, but a celebration of female sexuality. In the best of early neo burlesque performers of all ages, shapes and sizes clearly revelled in their bodies and performed their sexuality on their own terms. Certainly the shows of the early 1990s tended to be performed primarily for women, both gay and straight. While burlesque shows *can* be fun and affirming, if you haven't yet encountered this form of entertainment and are curious, I would choose your burlesque with some care. Sacrifice high end professionalism and go for a fringe show, rather than theatreland slick. 'Stripping classes' are sometimes run for women by burlesque performers, and here the emphasis will be firmly on fun rather than learning to be a performer.

'The stripping class was really good fun and the teacher was really encouraging and made me relaxed enough to go along with it all.'
Francoise 51, Print shop owner

I have been to a stripping class myself and while I had some reservations, it turned out to be tremendously enjoyable. Taught by a lovely and heavily pregnant burlesque professional, we learned to take off a glove with our teeth. It was an enormously mixed group of women of all ages and backgrounds and we all laughed ourselves silly. I wouldn't necessarily recommend this as a way to learn how to excite a partner, but I would *heartily* recommend it as an afternoon's fun with a friend or two. It was also rather good exercise!

References

Attwood, F. (2009) *Mainstreaming Sex: The sexualisation of Western Culture.* London: I. B. Tauris & Co Ltd.

Sex and the City, Season 1, Ep 9, *The Turtle and the Hare*, Aug 2, 1998.

1 2 3 4 5 6 7 8
9 10 11 12 13 14
15 16 17 18 19
20 **21 22 23 24**
25 26 27 28 29
30 31 32 33 34
35 36 37 38 39
40 41 42 43 44
45 46 47 48 49

Chapter 5

TALKING SEX, SHARING THE ADVENTURE

This chapter focuses on sexual communication, talking about sex in its widest sense. Of course, talking implies listening too, and that may mean listening to a partner, but also listening to what the wider world has to say about sexuality.

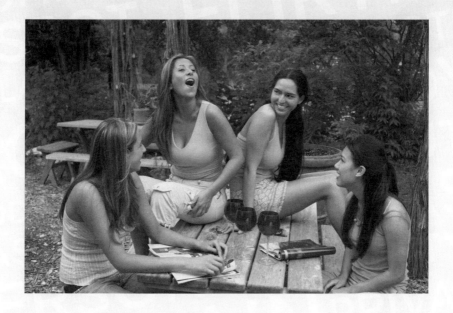

WAY 21 The importance of sexual communication

Most sex books will define sexual communication in terms of talking to a partner about our sexual desires or discussing our sexual relationship when things go wrong. We talk about both these things in Way 22 and Way 23. However, this is a book which takes a broader view of sexuality and which, I hope, has something to say about sexuality to everybody, whatever their relationship situation. Here, I want to discuss sexual communication in a wider sense.

Our quest for sexual well-being is one that takes us closer to becoming comfortable in our own sexuality. That notion of comfort incorporates being open to sexual communication – both in the sense of our own dialogue with others, but also in terms of our openness to being the recipients of sexual communication, to taking notice of sexual discussion in all sorts of contexts and from all sorts of sources. If, for whatever reason, we are struggling to see ourselves as sexual beings, then learning a few 'bedroom tricks' or buying a peep hole bra is only addressing the tip of the iceberg. Addressing our capacity for sexual communication is imperative in moving towards sexual self-actualisation. In other words, the woman who is comfortable with her sexuality is a woman who can comfortably (although of course *discriminatingly*) look at, think, read and talk about sex. You have already made a gesture towards sexual communication by buying this book. The format of the *49 Ways to Well-being* series facilitates communication, in that all individual Ways are short enough to share with a friend and make ideal jumping off points for further discussion.

My friend Ginny has been in a 'women's group' for many years. For her this has provided a forum in which to share feelings and ideas about all sorts of things, this is what she says:

'Over the years my women's group has been a lifeline. We are all very different, but it's also amazing how much we share experiences of bringing up children, coping with relationships, work difficulties and overall that constant juggling that women have to do every day. Recently one of my women started to talk about how she feels about her sexuality as she is getting older...we all started revealing our feelings about our increasingly sagging bodies, raging or otherwise libidos and our feelings about having sex with long term partners. We didn't all feel the same about things but it was fascinating, one of the best meetings we've ever had!'
Ginny 37, Librarian

Try this to gently bring sexual communication into your life – from all directions!:

- Try reading a novel which deals with sexual matters – see Way 14 for some suggestions. A sexy novel will always spark discussion – something for the book group perhaps?

- Look again at Way 14 for ideas about films which again may prove a useful discussion topic with friends or partner.

- Go to see an exhibition which deals with sexual themes – better still go with a friend so you can talk about it. Obviously it depends where you are and what's currently on, but you can bet that Sarah Lucas and Tracey Emin will always inspire heated debate around women and sexuality.

- If talking to friends about your feelings around sex feels daunting, try an online forum. The anonymity of online discussion may be a useful way to expand your sexual communication horizons and act as a precursor to a real life discussion.

Discussing and being open about our sexuality with others, as long as the setting is appropriate of course, is an important step in opening ourselves up to the possibility that sex may play a significant part in our lives. While it is always instructive and may often be comforting to share sexual confidences, it also goes without saying that, that sex is also funny at times. The many sexual situations in which we find ourselves can be awkward or even embarrassing but sharing these stories with friends can help to break down barriers and overcome obstacles to open sexual communication.

'We've all had times when sex goes wrong, we wear our best sexy underwear and try to look alluring and then fart in the middle of a passionate moment. The best thing about it is telling the story to our friends later after a few drinks, it helps doesn't it? Just to know that everyone's been there, sex shouldn't be serious and solemn all the time.
Vanessa 51 Teaching Assistant

WAY 22 Talking about your sexual needs

Undoubtedly, at times talking about one's sexual needs can be very difficult. Telling a partner what you want or desire in the context of a sexual relationship inevitably means exposing yourself at a very deep level, and when we are already exposing our physical selves, revealing our psyches as well may feel a step too far. Often our desires run counter to how we appear or want to represent ourselves in everyday life, for example, the successful and assertive women who longs to be subordinate sexually. Even quite simple requests can be hard to make; we are worried about turning our partner off or making demands that our partners find unstimulating or at worst distasteful.

At the start of a relationship talking about sex is a part of getting to know each other. Couples tend to share sexual experiences, likes and dislikes as a means to consolidating intimacy. However, we may have been in a relationship for a while and got into a rut, where sex is alright but not as satisfying as it could be. Asking for something new risks upsetting a partner who thinks everything is pretty much okay.

In a long term relationship problems may seem entrenched and dialogue might feel impossible to initiate, while at the other end of the scale our sex lives may simply be buried at the bottom of the laundry basket, just like that linen t-shirt you don't get round to putting in the machine because it means reading the washing instructions! If breaking the silence feels alarming rather than simply hard work, then I suggest you move to Way 23. If it has more in common with the fancy t-shirt that requires hand washing, let's think about how we might break this impasse.

Don't give up on improving the quality of sexual encounters. Many of us just end up going along with things rather than 'rocking the sexual boat', allowing our partner to dictate the pace and hoping that there will be time and stimulation enough for us to achieve satisfaction. In these scenarios often the love making ends when the man has ejaculated, leaving a partner to bring herself to orgasm. It's good to be assertive about what turns you on or off, but rather than issuing instructions during the act, which can test the confidence of any partner, try showing through your posture and the sounds you make what you are enjoying – ham it up a little! Most partners will be excited by your excitement. Move their hand gently and caressingly to where you want to be touched. 'Do as you would be done by' is a useful aphorism for sexual encounters!

- Try watching a sexy film together, it doesn't have to be hardcore (see some suggestions in Way 14). Making a positive suggestion such as, 'Ooh I'd really like to try that, that's a real turn on' may be exciting for a partner, rather than a threatening or critical 'Why don't we ever do that together?'.

- Turn your unspoken desires into a game over a glass or two of wine, along the lines of, 'I've always wanted to.... Your turn!'. Agree in advance that neither of you will be judgemental of the other's predilections, but will give something a go, unless it is a real turn-off for you. It might be useful to agree a sort of 'safe word' in advance which you can use to signal, without showing any distaste or disapproval, that you really do not want to experiment in that particular way.

Outside of the actual sexual act, it is vital to take any notion of blame or resentment out of conversations about sex with a partner. Keeping things as light hearted as possible is also a way to help ensure that neither party feels 'got at' or inadequate.

Relationships will suffer from misunderstandings and poor sexual communication around sex from time to time. I have experienced being locked into a spiral of sexual deterioration in which neither my partner or I could see beyond the idea that individually, we were not getting what we needed. The resulting antagonism, disappointment and damaged self-confidence only exacerbates mutual problems. What I have found most helpful is for each of us to step back from our own resentments and try to listen to the other without judging, responding with our own emotional reactions or imposing our own interpretation on what has been said. It is this effort to acknowledge and accept difference in terms of sexuality, sexual response and sexual expectations which is likely to be most fruitful in mending a sometimes fraught sexual life. That doesn't mean that one can always be (or *want* to deliver) what the other partner needs but recognising another's perspective can help us to move out of that quagmire of poor sexual communication.

WAY 23
Ways to approach talking about sex when things are difficult

When sex seems a thing of the distant past, or has become perfunctory and unsatisfying, discussing what's happening between you and a partner can sometimes lead to a problem becoming even more entrenched. When a problem is framed as *belonging* to one or other of you, then you are bound to start any conversation off on the wrong foot. Either partner can end up feeling pigeonholed in a particular role in relation to your sexual life, for example, one may be seen as the pursuer or aggressor who '*always* wants sex', while the other is the 'refuser' or 'avoider' who *never* wants it. These stereotypes are never helpful and can bolster and re-enforce an existing area of difficulty.

When talking about sex, also try to avoid over exaggerating the problem. Using phrases such as 'You never' or 'You always' are likely to turn what may be a temporary glitch into a self-fulfilling prophesy. Instead, try approaching discussion from a more positive perspective, talking about your sexual life together, rather than focusing on your feelings of hurt or anger towards each other.

- Try to envisage what your ideal sex life would look like. If you have been together for 10 years it is unlikely to be intense and passionate all the time, and presenting a partner with an overly idealised image of sexual bliss may feel like yet more pressure. While, of course, there may be the odd erotic encounter behind the kitchen island, perhaps relaxed, fun and experimental sex might be a more credible aim! Talk to your partner about how you would like your sex life to be, ensuring that you take the focus off what you would like *him* or *her* to *do* or *be*. Then ask your partner to imagine how they would like your sexual relationship to look and feel.

WAY 24 Talking about sex with friends

We live in an increasingly sexualised society in which commoditised sex confronts us at every turn. While our local community centre is running pole dancing classes, every stand-up comedian seems compelled to share (usually his) experiences of cunnilingus with an audience trying hard to look blasé, and 10-year-old girls are being exhorted to buy pencil cases bearing the Playboy bunny, it seems to me that we still have trouble talking to each other about our personal feelings around sexuality.

Sharing your feelings about sex with friends can be enormously therapeutic and often instructive. More importantly perhaps it can be fun, funny and enlightening. As in any other aspect of daily life, sharing experiences, concerns or ideas with others can open you up to new thinking as well as being a source of comfort or reassurance.

'Sex is funny, and the drama and dilemmas that go with it can be incredibly bonding. And it can be reassuring to talk about it. It's interesting to hear what other people find a turn on, but predominantly very funny!'
Eliza 48, Masseuse

Of course, it is far too easy to make assumptions about other people's relationships or what part sexuality plays in their lives. The cliché is that everybody imagines everyone else to be having a more active or satisfying sex life than they are themselves, and no doubt some people are swinging from rather more chandeliers than you are. However, if you are spending every night listening to your neighbours grunt and groan, don't assume that it is just luck or innate compatibility which has led to their energetic sex lives. Just possibly, if you have the sort of relationship which can stand a little self-exposure on both sides, they can give you a tip or two about how they prioritise or make space for sex in their lives. One of the gifts of sex talk is the unexpected revelation – the seemingly straight-laced friend who harbours surprising fantasies, the youthful experiences of your elderly parents – these things can remind us to acknowledge the centrality of sexuality to everyone's life.

In our concern not to invade people's privacy, and to be empathic and sensitive, I feel that we sometimes forget that talking about sex is just as entertaining as watching the latest blockbuster – quite possibly far more so. What's more, when you are scrabbling to recover the sexual persona that eludes you, talking about sex is really *de rigueur*! *Being* sexual requires you to *represent* yourself as sexual, and so a certain amount of openness or willingness to discuss sexual matters is part and parcel of moving towards the sexually self-actualised you. Don't take it all too seriously and, if this is something you feel nervous about, then start small!

Try some other ways to introduce sex as a topic of conversation with friends:

- Introduce a conversation with friends about best or worst sex scenes in books or films. This means that you don't have to reveal more of your personal feelings or experiences than you feel you want to.

- Open up a conversation by going shopping in one of the new women-only sex shops with a friend (see Way 17). Alternatively, a 'pampering' session (ghastly phrase for something quite enjoyable!) at a beauty salon or spa, lingerie shopping, or just a 'girls night' might be a setting that facilitates conversation that strays towards the intimate or risqué.

- If you feel confident enough, then put a toe in the water and ask women friends about their most *sensual* experience. Make it clear that you are not talking about actual sexual encounters. Try turning this into a game over drinks or at a dinner party with close friends: how about doing it alphabetically – 'What was your most sensual experience beginning with…', 'g' for gloves, for example.

WAY 25

Discussing your sexuality with a professional

Everybody has sexual difficulties at some point. While the constant presence of sexual representation bombarding us via all forms of media may lead us to conclude that everyone else's sex lives are not only successful but adventurous, experimental and passionate, this in itself creates an additional pressure on relationships that may be feeling a little stretched. Problems can arise at any point in a relationship, and it may be that difficulties in your sexual relationship feel so deep-rooted that addressing them alone seems a Herculean task. If this is the situation you are in, it is worth considering going to see a sex and relationship therapist.

Some people may have anxieties about taking up this sort of therapy. Perhaps these anxieties centre on what will happen during the sessions, what the sex therapist will be like or whether problems are not 'bad enough' (or 'too bad'!) for treatment. Firstly, sex therapy is simply another 'talking therapy', a branch of traditional psychotherapy or counselling. It has the same sort of format as any other talking therapy, for example, it will take place in an ordinary room and you will *never* be asked to do anything physical except in the privacy of your own home. Secondly, the therapist is very unlikely to be a 'dippy hippy' in the Barbara Streisand *Meet the Fockers* mould (although I confess to a real fondness for that character) and will never impose his or her own moral values on your behaviour. Finally, if your difficulties are getting in the way of a satisfying sex life or causing emotional distress, then therapy is an avenue worth thinking about. Just finding out how common a difficulty is may help move you towards a solution. It is always better to address problems before they become deeply entrenched. A sex therapist will recognise that most people who have sought a sex therapist are finding it difficult to discuss sexual matters. Often, feelings of anger, hurt, inhibition or disappointment get in the way of really productive discussion between a couple, and this is the situation in which a trained third party is invaluable. The therapist will provide a safe and non-judgemental environment, help you to feel comfortable discussing your sexual issues, and gently guide your discussion by creating a positive framework which allows you to unravel problems together.

See the Further Information, Reading and Resources section to this chapter for suggestions on where to go for sex therapy.

1 2 3 4 5 6 7 8
9 10 11 12 13 14
15 16 17 18 19
20 21 22 23 24
25 **26 27 28 29
30** 31 32 33 34
35 36 37 38 39
40 41 42 43 44
45 46 47 48 49

Chapter 6

MYTHS AND MAGIC: FEMALE AROUSAL

This chapter gets down to some of the fundamentals of female pleasure and arousal, but starts by thinking about how we characterise male and female pleasure differently. Here, we start by asking whether constructing male and female sexuality as different is helpful in terms of our personal journey of sexual discovery.

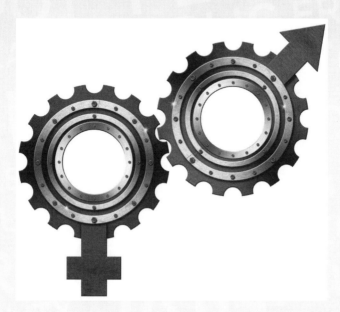

26 Feminine sexuality/ male sexuality

The idea that male and female sexuality is intrinsically different is widespread. In Western societies the stereotypical view is that men are more 'highly sexed' or have a more 'functional' attitude to sex than women. Men are traditionally thought to be focused primarily on the sexual act, viewing it as a sort of itch that needs to be scratched, whereas women are said to have a more emotional experiencing of sex, understanding it in the context of feelings and relationships. The prevalence of these ideas underlines the notion that men are the primary users of pornography. However, recent research of 5,490 pornography users suggests that, while overall more men than women are viewing porn, the picture is changing and younger women show more interest in porn than older women. Possibly over time these differences in porn use by men and women will even out: this is evidenced not least by developments in the availability of women-friendly pornography (see Way 15). While these so called 'differences' dominate the way we talk about gender when it comes to sexuality, it is important to remember that ideas about male and female sexuality vary hugely across different historical periods and within different cultures. Furthermore, research that appears to prove gendered differences in the way we think about sex, or what gets men and women aroused, has always been countered by other research which 'proves' no such differences exist.

'I have to be slipping in and out of a coma not to feel sexy. They say men think about sex every few minutes. I think women, particularly as they get older, are completely in charge, they know what they want and they go and get it.'
Eliza 48, Masseur

These ideas about how men and women feel about sex are nothing more than stereotypes, and stereotypes can get in the way or even prevent us understanding and exploring our own sexual worlds. Even now, if a woman is forthright and assertive sexually, she may find that she is perceived as threatening by others; she may be seen to be distorting a natural order of things in which the man is the more highly sexualised partner and, therefore, the one who takes the initiative in sexual scenarios. Those women who are open in talking about themselves in the context of their sexual interests may be given a number of disparaging and belittling labels: slut, cougar, laddette, party girl and so on. Sadly the polarisation of women into 'good girls' and 'bad girls' is still very prevalent and those like Amy (below) who like sex and enjoy discussing it, may be seen as exhibiting inappropriate behaviour in social situations.

'I have always found it difficult to be myself sexually. Because I am open in talking about sex and interested in the subject, others, both men and women, see me as oversexed and make a joke about how I'm always going on about sex. I find it difficult to express myself and I think people misunderstand me and just see me as some sort of "up for it" woman, but that's not what it's about for me.'
Amy 47, Social worker

Continuing widespread pressures around women and sexuality force us to present ourselves in ways deemed acceptable by our social group. As women reach middle age, my feeling is that women's outlets for sexual self-expression become even more limited and women, whether introverted or extraverted in their approach to sexuality, are occupied by appearing in ways which don't rock the boat.

- How do you feel you currently present yourself to others in terms of your sexuality? Are you someone who acts on your sexual urges or are you more reserved, tending to hold back? Do you enjoy talking frankly about sexual matters or are you a private person when it comes to discussing sex?

- Once you have managed to define your sexual style in a way that feels accurate and comfortable to you, note to yourself how many opportunities you have to be that person and who in your social circle you feel able to be that person with. It may be that if you are anxious about how you appear to others – whether open and forthright or reticent and reserved – you are opening the door to criticism and attracting judgmental people. A woman who is accepting of herself and feels comfortable 'in her own skin' naturally communicates this to the people around her, attracting those who are accepting and supportive.

This book has repeatedly emphasised the idea of sexuality as not being only about sex, or 'doing it', as it were. It is important that a woman finds a way of being comfortable with her own sexuality and opportunities to express and explore her sexual nature outside of the constraints of gender stereotypes. These opportunities may not be within the confines of a relationship and are not necessarily simply about performing the sex act. Here we are concerned primarily about ways to *be* and that may involve talking, reading, watching, shopping and so on (see Ways 14, 15, 16, 17, 21, 24).

Orgasm: clitoris versus vagina

'I never understood the point of debating about orgasms: you have them, they're great. Probably no two are ever exactly the same but embrace the variety I say!'
Asma 34 , Local council worker

Whether there is a difference between a clitoral and vaginal orgasm, whether or not women experience vaginal orgasms at all and which is better if they do, is still the subject of much debate and has been for decades. Freud's assertion that focus on the clitoris is somehow indicative of an immature sexuality has had a far reaching influence which has shaped much of our current thinking about the clitoris/vagina debate. Shere Hite suggested in the Hite Report of 1976 that 70% of us don't orgasm this way. In what remains a highly controversial piece of research, Hite made the very significant point that cultural and social assumptions about the nature of 'normal' female sexuality will impact on the outcome of research. Her own research strongly refuted that having an orgasm during coitus was 'normal', yet this is a notion that women still wrestle with today and it still plays a large part in women's everyday experience of sex with a male partner. Perhaps the only conclusion to draw from the volumes of heated discussion down the decades is that women experience orgasm differently in terms of both where it is and what it feels like; our understanding of what an orgasm is, is largely that – an understanding.

In the long run it doesn't matter, it may not even matter to you whether or not you experience orgasm with a partner. What *is* important, however, is that you experience sex as pleasurable. But what I do want to emphasise here is that you do not orgasm in a vacuum; your orgasm, whether it is vaginal, clitoral or because you've stuck a cotton bud in your left ear, has been argued over, commoditised and represented in a myriad ways. It is not easy to discover what *you* need to become aroused and sexually satiated, when that necessarily involves finding your way through decades of assumption, political debate, rampant sexual commercialism, media speculation and the impact all this has on the intimate sexual negotiations that go on between sexual partners. All in all, this is a good argument for getting to know your body and what turns *you* on in order that you can explain your preferences and gently guide a partner to facilitate your pleasure.

'I know lots of women say they can't orgasm through penetrative sex but I do orgasm vaginally, almost every time. I think I'm just lucky because of where my clitoris is positioned, it gets stimulated by the friction of my husband's penis when we have sex, it must be high up or something, it's never been a problem for me. I masturbate to orgasm to help me get to sleep quite a lot too, I have a problem with not sleeping and I find this a useful way to make myself sleepy. On the whole I don't experience any difference between giving myself an orgasm and having an orgasm through sex with my partner.'

Pam 29, Trainee midwife

Orgasm checklist. You will need:

- complete privacy and no time constraints
- somewhere comfortable to be: a bed, bath or wherever you are unlikely to be disturbed
- some sort of fantasy material which could be generated by your own imagination or by an external source (see Chapter 3)
- some sort of implement, I suggest a finger but see Chapter 4 for alternative suggestions!

You will *also* need:

- to be aware of the overarching importance of exploring your sexuality to your own health and well-being
- an understanding that orgasm can help you unwind after a stressful day, induce sleep when you are locked in a cycle of anxious thoughts, and help relieve pain, for example nagging joint or back pain
- a complete absence of guilt, unless of course guilt is part of your fantasy!

28 When the flame becomes a flicker

Perhaps you have picked up this book because you feel your sexual energy is depleted or you fear that you are not enjoying sex with your partner as much as you could or are *supposed* or *expected* to. When you are fumbling to locate your sex drive amidst the dust balls and lost socks underneath that sideboard, it is vital to examine where the root of the problem might be.

Body worries can be a major source of inhibition around sexuality. Conscious or unconscious fears that our body is unattractive in some way can be a major stumbling block to enjoying sex with a partner. Focusing on how your body looks to someone else can be enormously distracting as well as limiting in terms of exploration and experimentation, for example, if you are convinced your body only looks acceptable if you are lying on your back! I believe strongly in the power of seeing ordinary bodies. Every day we are faced with young adult bodies, retouched to mimic perfection – the relief of seeing real bodies in a swimming pool changing room can be immense and allow us to be more accepting of ourselves.

Feeling under pressure to orgasm or even to show excitement can be a killer. The male orgasm obviously results in a very conspicuous climax, we can't really miss it and because of this there is a danger that the male orgasm becomes the main focus of the sexual act. What's more, over recent years we have been hearing more and more about what is known as female ejaculation (see Way 30), yet another milestone to be notched up on the road to being seen as a truly sexual woman. If a woman feels under pressure, not only to ensure that her partner is satisfied, but to make her own multi-faceted sexual ecstasy visible in order to ensure another's pleasure, then sex can feel like simply going through the motions – primarily for someone else's gratification.

Look at the box opposite. See Chapter 5 for more thoughts on communicating with a partner about these and other sexual matters. If talking about your needs feels really difficult, it may well be useful to visit a sex therapist for support in finding your way back to mutually satisfying sex (see Way 25).

- Try taking penetrative sex out of the equation by banning it for a few weeks. If you can, talk to your partner about how you are feeling, explain that the attempt to reach orgasm this way is distracting you from enjoying other wonderful sexual sensations. This approach is based on what is known as 'sensate focus'. Conceived by Masters and Johnson, it involves a gradual move (over some weeks) from initial non-sexual touching between partners to increasingly sexualised caresses. Try to make sure that this strategy doesn't come across as an implied criticism of your partner's technique or expectations. If both partners commit to giving this a try, it can be a positive move towards not only experiencing sex more fully but also building up a bit of sexual energy between you – forbidding a particular or familiar element of your sexual repertoire can be a fun way to finding your way back to sexual pleasure! For fuller guidance on how to use the sensate focus technique, try http://counselling-matters.org.uk/sites/counselling-matters/files/SensateFocus.pdf

- For many of us, coitus is not the route to sexual satisfaction but that doesn't mean that it can't be an enjoyable part of sexual practice. It may be that you need your partner to bring you to orgasm manually, with a toy, or his or her tongue. Perhaps sometimes (or most of the time), you prefer to bring yourself to orgasm but would like your partner to participate in some other way, by telling you a sexy story or just by holding you while you climax. It makes me fume that most visual representations of the sex act still show the woman climaxing through intercourse; this is a construction of sex which prioritises the needs of a male partner and one which effectively puts enormous pressure on women to perform in a very particular way, possibly involving the sublimation of her own sexual needs.

29 Spot the G spot

Sometimes it can feel as if the whole G spot debate is something like a highly sophisticated version of *Where's Wally!* Where is it? Does it exist at all? What if you can't find it? Will locating my G spot make me a more sexual woman? The G spot first came to our attention in 1982, when sexologists Ladas, Whipple and Perry published a bestselling book called *The G-Spot and Other Discoveries About Human Sexuality*. They named this area of the vaginal wall the 'G spot' after Dr Ernst Grafenberg, who had been the first to describe *The Role of the Urethra in Female Orgasm* in 1950. The claim is that stimulation of this area may result in sexual arousal, more potent orgasms and possibly female ejaculation (more on this later).

The existence of the G spot has been much argued over. While science has failed to find convincing and sustained evidence that it exists, many women do maintain that it has a role to play in female sexual pleasure. Inevitably, the debate has been taken up by the popular press and over the past three decades much copy has been generated around how to find it and what it does. Furthermore, it has been commoditised in the form of a myriad vibrators and dildos which claim to offer G spot delight: many vibrators have probes aimed at stimulating the clitoris, the G spot and the vagina – a sort of 'try everything' approach (see Way 19). While all this may have led to some women discovering a new source of sensation, for others it has engendered a sense of failure if they can't find it or can't see what all the fuss is about. Furthermore, some feminists would say that talk about the G spot is part of a conspiracy to re-establish the vaginal orgasm, arrived at through penetrative sex with a male partner, as the primary goal of sexual activity. Any cursory glance at the results of an internet search for G spot will show just how much confusion and debate is still rife concerning it.

- The G spot, sometimes known as the 'female prostate' because it is said to contain tiny prostate style glands, is purported to be between one and three inches inside the front (anterior) of the vaginal wall.

- You don't need to buy a piece of rotating pink plastic to find it or to stimulate it. If you put a finger inside your vagina, palm upwards and make a beckoning motion you may find a slightly ridged area which feels a bit like the area of your mouth behind your front teeth – if you do, this is apparently the G spot.

- Try experimenting with different sex positions; one or other may serve to successfully stimulate your G spot. Many women find that being on top allows them control over the angle at which the penis enters and presses on their vaginal wall – the missionary position may not be the best for G spot stimulation – see Gabriella's testimony below.

- It may be that, once aroused, if you press on this area, you will feel an increased level of arousal or experience a more powerful orgasm (I'm afraid nothing much is likely to happen if you have not achieved a level of arousal already). On the other hand you may feel as if you want to do a wee. Try it and see!

'I'm not really sure whether or not it's to do with the G Spot, I'm not entirely sure about that, but I do find that some positions give me a more intense sensation, are far more arousing – for me anyway. I think it must be to do with the way the penis hits my vaginal wall or something. The missionary position does nothing for me, it's just a sensation of 'fullness', neither here nor there! What I like best is sex from behind – I hate that expression "doggy style". That position seems to stimulate my vagina in a different way and I think it must be because the penis is pushing against my G Spot. Well, whatever it is, it works for me!'
Gabriella 45, Dental Technician

30 Female ejaculation and other high points!

Like the existence and function of the G spot, so called 'female ejaculation' is something that inspires controversy and enthusiasm in equal measure. Variously discussed over centuries, it is said to be a fluid expelled from the urethra at or around the point of orgasm. Most of the debate is concerned with what it is made up of, with detractors suggesting that it is mainly urine, and supporters of the notion of female ejaculation saying that it is a watery liquid that originates in the female prostate. The porn industry has been enthusiastic in its take up of the idea that women, like men, produce ejaculate. Undoubtedly, this is because any visible representation of sexual excitement is good news for screen based media and 'squirting' and 'gushing' have become terms embedded in pornographic dialogue. The British Board of Film Classification has banned films which purport to show female ejaculation on the basis that there is no substantial medical proof that this is anything but urination, and the combination of urination and sex is deemed to be obscene under British law. Feminist response to the idea that women ejaculate is divided along the lines of whether it signals empowerment or whether the whole notion of ejaculation is simply a masculine construction of sexuality being foisted onto women.

If there is a little more moisture on the sheets than usual after a sex session, don't worry, you could just say excitedly 'Oh look, I've ejaculated!'. No doubt your partner will be thrilled that he or she has inspired such transports of delight! The only thing that really concerns me here is that women do not use the idea of female ejaculation as yet another stick to beat themselves with – along the lines of, 'Do I or don't I and what does this say about me and my sexuality?' However, if you want to explore the idea, then the consensus seems to be that it is linked to the G spot: stimulation of the G spot during sex may or may not lead to ejaculation but it's worth a try just for fun!

You may be saying 'If it ain't broke don't fix it' at this point! However, here are some ideas to play with which may or may not intensify or prolong the orgasmic response.

- Delaying orgasm is a technique which is said to offer a heightened experience for some. Try letting your body reach a peak of excitement and then pause for a few seconds to let the peak subside a little. Keep on allowing yourself to reach the threshold of orgasm and then pausing before you get there. This technique is a good way to build tension, hopefully resulting in a more powerful orgasm. The drawback is that you may lose focus and orgasm may slip away.

- Try clenching and tensing your muscles in the stomach, thighs and rectum area as your pleasure intensifies and then let go to encourage your body to relax as you reach orgasm.

- Placing the soles of your feet together (bend your knees to create a diamond shape between your legs) is said to give a stronger orgasm – try it!

- Try orgasm with a moderately full bladder (may also help ejaculation – only kidding!). This creates pressure which may intensify the orgasmic experience.

- Strengthen your pelvic floor muscles; this is a good goal for all women particularly after childbirth and regardless of any sexual intention. However, it can also improve your experience of sex. Please note this is about your pleasure, not your ability to clamp your vagina around some masculine member! Try holding the pelvic floor muscle squeezed for a count of ten then relaxing, and repeat this action ten times. It is a good idea to do this at a particular point in the day or make some everyday activity a trigger for this exercise. Personally, I try to do it in the car whenever I get to some traffic lights!

References

Attwood, F. (2009) *Mainstreaming Sex: The sexualisation of Western Culture*. London: I. B. Taurus.

Ladas, A. K., Whipple, B. and Perry, J. D. (1982) *The G spot. And other discoveries about human sexuality*. New York: Holt, Rinehart and Winston.

1 2 3 4 5 6 7 8
9 10 11 12 13 14
15 16 17 18 19
20 21 22 23 24
25 26 27 28 29
30 **31 32 33 34**
35 36 37 38 39
40 41 42 43 44
45 46 47 48 49

Chapter 7

SEXUAL WELLNESS

Sometimes things are just difficult sexually speaking. This chapter explains some common challenges women may encounter, providing some pointers to moving things in a happier direction.

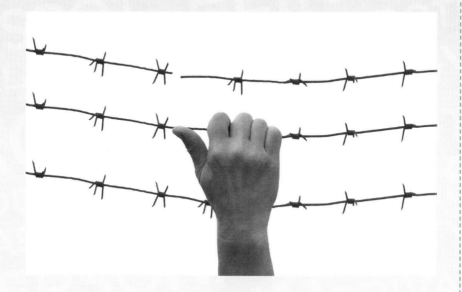

WAY 31 Sex and pain

Studies suggest that anything from 6 to 33 per cent of women experience significant pain during or after intercourse – depending, unsurprisingly, on who the researchers ask, what they ask, and how they ask it. Younger women in their 20s appear twice as susceptible as women in their 50s. In pinning down causes, doctors distinguish superficial dyspareunia – pain when the penis enters the vagina, from deep dyspareunia – deeper pelvic pain on thrusting.

Superficial pain generally arises from the vagina, and vaginismus (see Way 33) is one important cause. Another is atrophic vaginitis, loss of suppleness and lubrication of vaginal skin in women following their menopause, which usually responds well to treatment with hormone replacement therapy (HRT) or vaginal oestrogen cream or pessaries. Infections, particularly candida (thrush) or trichomonas, scarring following surgery such as episiotomy repair or female genital mutilation (FGM), vaginal dryness or simple lack of stimulation are also often implicated. A hymen that hasn't yet completely ruptured, together with anxiety and inexperience, often conspire to make first attempts at intercourse painful in young women.

- Foreplay until you're aroused, and have gentle sex with plenty of lube.

- Treat thrush symptoms such as soreness, itching, cheesy white discharge. Otherwise, see your doctor.

Deeper pain might be the result of pelvic infection, or endometriosis – a painful condition where fragments of womb lining migrate out into the pelvis to cause bleeding and scarring. About 80% of women have a womb which tilts forwards, and a backwards-tilting, retroverted uterus used to be considered a cause of painful sex. Nowadays that's regarded as unlikely unless other conditions are present, such as adhesions – scar tissue from previous infection or surgery. Ovaries usually lie beside your womb, but if one or both have moved (prolapsed) behind the womb, they can be squeezed painfully during sex.

- If you have a contraceptive coil fitted, check the threads – a low-lying device is another possible cause.
- Deep dyspareunia is often worse with certain sexual positions, so experiment. Otherwise, see your doctor.

Pain during orgasm isn't fully understood – one possibility is that it arises from cramp of the womb muscle, though some doctors suspect it might be a side-effect of some antidepressants or contraceptive pills.

- Experiment with sexual position, take a painkiller prior to sex, and check with your doctor if you're taking medication.

Pain *after* sex can have similar causes to deep pain during sex, though post-intercourse backache often points to a straightforward problem with the spine or back muscles, and cramps might suggest a bowel problem such as irritable bowel syndrome (IBS).

- Take painkillers before sex and experiment with sexual positions
- Ensure a high-fibre diet and keep your bowels regular.

Painful sex seems to improve on its own in around one-third of women, but a striking finding in confidential studies has been the low proportion of sufferers, around a quarter, who ever mention the problem to their doctor. Dyspareunia isn't generally likely to indicate anything serious or life-threatening, but depending on the cause, treatment with exercises, counselling, drugs or surgery could change your life.

- An appointment with your GP!

When things go wrong: anorgasmia

For women orgasm may be elusive, and furthermore, unlike the male orgasm, female climax may be difficult to identify – some women may be unable to say whether or not they have actually achieved orgasm. Supposedly 'objective' and medical indicators of orgasm have been argued about for decades. In his ground-breaking work *Sexual Behaviour in the Human Female* (1953), Alfred Kinsey offered one definition of it as the: 'cessation of the oft times strenuous movements and extreme tensions of the previous sexual activity and the peace of the resulting state'. Masters and Johnson in *Human Sexual Response* (1966) provide a definition that is more concise but possibly even more obtuse: 'a sensation of suspension or stoppage'. Physiological evidence-based indicators of orgasm include the labia becoming engorged and so increasing in size, as well as a deepening in colour, and a muscle contraction in the outer third of the vagina which lasts for some seconds.

Anorgasmia (or orgasmic disorder) is the word used to describe a state in which a woman is able to become sexually excited but unable to reach orgasm. Some women report a lack of orgasm over a period of time, in other words they have had orgasms but are not climaxing currently or only in particular circumstances, such as via masturbation (this is known as secondary orgasmic dysfunction). Occasionally however, women report that they have never experienced at orgasm at all in any situation or circumstances (primary orgasmic dysfunction).

Anorgasmia is usually treated by cognitive behavioural approaches focusing on reducing anxiety and changing thought patterns. Negative constructions of female sexuality or sex itself, as well as a habit of self-monitoring during sex, may interfere with women's ability to reach orgasm. Inevitably, past experience, particularly childhood experience and upbringing, may be implicated in lack of sexual response. Sometimes guilt may contribute to anorgasmia, for example, where the woman was brought up in a very religious or repressive environment for example. Masturbation may play a large part in helping those with orgasmic disorder. In masturbation, any anxiety connected with a partner is removed and excitement and hopefully climax is totally under the woman's control. It is important to separate anorgasmia from lack of desire or a reduced sex drive. Those who are unable to experience orgasm, whether it only appears to be a temporary state of affairs or whether it is deeper rooted, should seek professional help to address this problem (see Way 25).

33 Sexual dysfunction

Sexual dysfunction is usually defined as something that interferes with the performance of the sexual act (which typically tends to mean penetration by the male of the female). That, aside pain and dryness, can make even masturbation uncomfortable and vaginismus is of course enormously frustrating, distressing and not uncommon.

Dr Martin Edwards, a GP and writer on health issues, offers some information and advice on the topic of vaginismus:

The American gynaecologist J. Marion Sims first coined the term when he defined vaginismus in 1861, though plausible descriptions exist at least from the 16th century. Sims described 'an involuntary spasmodic closure of the mouth of the vagina, attended with such excessive supersensitiveness as to form a complete barrier to coition.' This rather loose clinical definition – vaginismus as involuntary spasm of vaginal muscles, and in extreme cases the inner thigh muscles, pulling the legs inseparably together – has persisted since, though has faced criticism for being subjective and lacking firm evidence. Nonetheless, attempted penetration with a penis, finger, or – in extreme cases – tampon is painful and frequently impossible, male partners describing the sensation of an impenetrable wall. Psychological explanations classically distinguish secondary vaginismus – which arises following a traumatic experience such as rape, or painful conditions such as episiotomy scarring – from the more common primary vaginismus, present from puberty or before, which might follow abuse or repressive sexual upbringing. More recent theories prioritise fear, regarding vaginismus as akin to a type of penetration phobia. The loose definition of the condition, and reluctance of many women to seek help, make it difficult to gauge just how common it is, though most estimates suggest that vaginismus affects around ten per cent of adult women – making it one of the most common disorders of sexual function. Fortunately, therapy is generally regarded as highly effective. Sims originally advocated surgery, which was largely replaced with psychotherapeutic approaches by the mid-twentieth century. Treatment nowadays generally involves the gentle insertion of vaginal dilators of steadily increasing size, though psychological treatments, drugs such as local anaesthetics or muscle relaxants (including botulinum toxin or botox injections), pelvic relaxation techniques and couple-based sex therapy, all claim success.

Vaginal dryness is distinct from vaginismus, but either condition might provoke the other. Around half of all postmenopausal women experience problems due to atrophic vaginitis – soreness, dryness and ultimately even shrinkage of their vaginal skin, arising from reduced levels of the oestrogen hormone responsible for keeping vaginal skin supple and lubricated. Usually it's easily treated with hormone replacement therapy, or oestrogen cream or pessaries applied to the vagina. Less attention tends to be paid to vaginal dryness in younger women, though it remains an under-reported problem probably experienced by around five per cent of women in the UK. Causes can be hormonal (pregnancy, breastfeeding, surgery to remove ovaries), rarities such as Sjogren's syndrome which affects moisture-producing cells, or the side-effects of drugs including contraceptives, decongestants and antidepressants. But probably most common is simply anxiety, tension or a lack or arousal.

Use a proprietary moisturiser for everyday comfort, and a lubricant for sex – some preparations can do both jobs, but generally they're designed for one or the other. Some lubricants can damage condoms – read the instructions.

Don't skimp on foreplay, it helps you relax and become aroused. Ask your doctor about any medication you're taking.

WAY 34

Sex and mental health: depression and SSRIs

Sexuality is not just the means by which we re-produce ourselves; it is an instinct which guides much of our behaviour and helps to define us. This book has stressed the idea that sexuality is not limited to ideas around attraction, nor is it necessarily about having sex. We have focused on sexuality as an attribute of our individuality, as a matter of how we perceive ourselves and present ourselves to others. If we are out of tune with ourselves as sexual beings, if we deny our sexuality or repress it, if we lack confidence in expressing ourselves as sexual beings in our daily lives, then ultimately our mental health will be affected.

On the other hand, it is also true to say that depression, anxiety and other mental health difficulties can impact on our capacity to enjoy sex or to see ourselves as sexual agents. Lack of interest in sex is one of the key indicators of depression. It is very common indeed for sex to go out of the window when we are coping with life's difficulties; illness, loss, divorce, work problems and so on may easily push our sexuality to the bottom of the pile or turn sex into a chore – yet another thing to worry about. It is clear that this can become a circular problem. 'Life is overwhelming, I don't have space or time to feel sexual', yet 'I don't feel sexual anymore and that makes me feel low about myself'.

Poor sex drive can be a side effect of medication taken for mental health problems such as depression and anxiety. Whether or not lack of libido is due to the medication itself may be difficult to determine in individual cases because depression itself often impacts on sexual feelings. However, it does seem to be fairly well established that many so called SSRI type anti-depressants (for example Fluoxetine, commonly known as Prozac) may have a detrimental effect on both sexual function and sexual enjoyment. Why this should be is not yet well understood by the medical profession, but SSRIs can induce or exacerbate difficulties such as erectile dysfunction in men, lack of arousal, inability to experience orgasm or poor quality orgasms. If you are taking an anti-depressant and experiencing sexual problems, it is worth talking this over with your GP who may be able to prescribe an alternative medication less associated with this kind of side effect.

'I suffer from intermittent but long term depression and anxiety. When I'm feeling poorly, sex is the last thing on my mind and the idea of feeling sexual just seems like a cruel joke, you know what I mean? But recently I've realized that this contributes to my feeling a lack of self-worth at these times – I stop looking after myself, stop seeing myself as a sexual woman and then I end up feeling worse about myself than ever. Now I try to do small things to look after myself, like eating a good meal or making sure I'm taking care with what I'm wearing. I know I sound like an advert but it's like saying 'I am worth it'!'

Vanessa 51, Teaching assistant

Take care of your sexual self. Losing touch with our sexuality can impact negatively on both our physical and mental sense of well-being, if sexuality is a part of our identity it is also a part of how we express ourselves and how we interact with others.

It can help just to view looking after our sexuality as a form of self-care. Just as when you are struggling to maintain or improve your mental health, it is important to look after your needs in terms of eating good nutritious food at regular intervals, to focus on structuring your day and to take regular exercise (enormously valuable in boosting your endorphin levels), so it is vital to maintain your sexual self at times of stress.

Looking after your sexual self might include ensuring you are well dressed and groomed, using some special body lotion after a bath, ensuring your home is sensually appealing by buying yourself some flowers. When our ability to be kind to ourselves is challenged, these small acts work as validations of the importance we attach to keeping ourselves well. To take this one stage further, consider a little gentle flirting (see Way 7). Practising your flirting techniques on the man in the corner shop may give you a much needed boost and help to remind you that you are more than the sum of your problems.

WAY 35 Sex and disability

While the word 'sexuality' is often associated with 'having sex', in this book we have been working towards a far broader definition; sexuality is about our identity, our sexual orientation, the roles we play, our fantasies, desires and our practices. Furthermore, sexuality and the way we express our sexuality is not simply an individual choice or expression of selfhood, it is influenced by social factors, class, economics and politics.

It goes without saying that all of us, whatever our shape, size, background, culture, gender, disability, and so on, experience desires, pleasures, doubts and worries when it comes to sexuality and our sex lives. Sex is something that will trip all of us up at some point in our lives! Similarly, difference is inevitable; we all have bodies that are different – bodies that look, smell and taste different from other bodies. There may be particular *parts* of our bodies that we focus on as different. Sometimes, given the panoply of 'perfection' we are faced with every day via a multiplicity of media channels, we forget what all our bodies have in common – for example, our internal or reproductive organs may be exactly the same as most women's. The fact that our body looks different does not mean that it is deficient in any way.

Sadly, many people find sex and sexuality a difficult topic when it comes to people with disabilities. While most people with a disability can count on being supported to achieve a level of autonomy in every other aspect of their lives, services, governments, support workers and even the most enlightened of parents of disabled children or teenagers may tend to treat disabled people as if they are asexual. The widespread myths and stereotypes around disabled people and sexuality serve to make it difficult for those with disabilities to exercise their human sexual rights. As a result, people's access to sexual expression can sometimes be impeded by 'well meaning' safeguarding legislation as well as laws around sex work.

The website www.sexualityanddisability.org lists several key areas of myth-making around sexuality and disability: firstly, the idea that women with disabilities don't need sex. For the disabled woman it is often the assumptions and stereotypes around the topic of disability which get in the way of her experiencing her sexuality fully, rather than anything to do with their disability. Secondly, the notion that women with disabilities are not sexually attractive. What does it say about our society if all but the eighteen year old, size 8 model in *Vogue* is dismissed as not sexually attractive? Thirdly, women with disabilities have more pressing needs that those around sexuality. A disabled woman is often seen in terms of her basic needs – food, sleep, movement and so on – while the central and fundamental importance of sexuality to all people may be overlooked in the effort to meet those needs. Finally, www.sexualityanddisability.org debunks another myth which struck me as having resonance for all of us, whether disabled or able bodied. Sex does not need to be spontaneous:

'Women with disabilities may need to take some extra factors into account before having a sexual encounter with someone. She may need to think about the times of day when pain or tiredness are less of a problem, put a waterproof cover on the bed in case her bladder leaks, or may simply need to ensure that she has the privacy she desires. However, this doesn't make the sex women with disabilities have any less "natural" or "real" than those who don't have similar considerations.'

Unsurprisingly, the internet has enabled many people to pursue a fulfilling sex life. For many it has proved to be a highly successful means of finding a partner; it can also facilitate people in meeting specialist sexual needs, as well as allow anyone, whether disabled or able bodied, to indulge in online fantasy fulfillment. There is a wealth of information available on the topic of sexuality and disability, and I have listed some resources in the Further Information, Reading and Resources section to this chapter that I have found to be particularly helpful or informative.

References

Kinsey, A. *et al* (1953) *Sexual Behaviour in the Human Female*

Notes

1 2 3 4 5 6 7 8
9 10 11 12 13 14
15 16 17 18 19
20 21 22 23 24
25 26 27 28 29
30 31 32 33 34
35 **36 37 38 39
40** 41 42 43 44
45 46 47 48 49

Chapter 8

THE SEXUAL SELF AT DIFFERENT LIFE STAGES

Inevitably, our experience of sex varies at different times over the course of our lives. However, sometimes it is difficult to see just what stays the same, what has improved or what might be re-kindled. We all measure our lives through significant events – marriage, divorce, the birth of a child and so on – but lurking underneath these public milestones is another history – our sexual history. This intimate narrative is one that usually remains hidden in personal memory, but our first Way suggests that it can be useful to us today to shine a light on our sexual past.

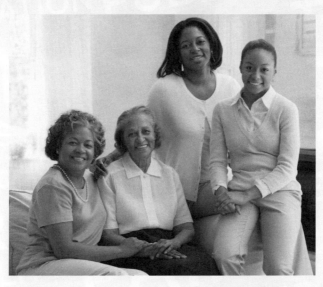

36 Sex through the ages

We are all guilty of peddling stereotypes around sex and our sexuality at different life stages. The young are lithe and lissom and have carefree, hedonistic, experimental sex. The middle aged have settled into dull routine, they 'know what they like' and have it regularly on a Saturday morning. The old don't have it at all.

Of course we also know that this is nonsense. If we're lucky, in our youth, we may have the odd sexual experience untroubled by anxiety and angst, but we will have other times when we are beset by worries about our attractiveness, how much our partner actually likes us, what other people think about our latest sexual exploit, and inevitably, not getting pregnant or acquiring a sexually transmitted disease. Middle age can be a time to experiment sexually, at ease in the security of a loving long term relationship. Alternatively, it may be a time when we are excited by the prospect of forging a new sexual identity; we may be trying out potential new partners and new sexual experiences. In later life all of the above may apply – possibly minus the pregnancy fears!

When we are feeling a little lost in terms of our sexual identity, when we feel our sexual selves are hidden in the mists of time, when our sex lives are at something of an impasse, it is easy to believe that there have been other life stages in which our sexuality was more assured, our sex lives more spontaneous, when sex was trouble free.

As in many areas of our life, it is useful to get all this into perspective. It may be helpful to spend a little time thinking about our sexuality at different life stages, asking questions such as 'What was my sex life like then?' 'What did that give me?' 'How did I feel about myself then?'

- Roughly, on paper – in order to give your thoughts a little structure – divide your life into 'chunks'. This will be different for everybody, because each person will see their life as having different distinct stages. For example, I would start with my late teens and early twenties, then early parenthood, moving into my late thirties and early forties and so on!

- Allocate each period three columns; you will adapt this as you go along and you might end up with several columns, but this is a good start.

- The first column will represent the sex life you were having (and importantly not having) during this time of your life: Who were you having it with or not? Where were you? What else occupied you at this time of your life?

- The second and third columns should focus on you. As far as you can remember, jot down your beliefs and feelings about yourself at that time in relation to your sexuality. One column will represent positive feelings and the other negative – there may be cross-overs here but that's good.

- Keep going until you are up to date and have reached your life now.

The aim here is simply to help us look at our sexual lives without the interference of either a golden haze or a grey mist. We may see patterns, for example, the exercise may show that our sexual self-confidence soared at times when we were without a long term partner, or that it dipped in our early 20s when we have always believed we were at our most attractive. Looking at our sexual past and recalling how we read and understood ourselves in relation to sexual experience, can help us to break the habits of unhelpful stereotyping which hold us back today.

Look back at Ways 21 and 24, which are about talking and sharing with others. This can be a powerful conversation to have with friends, old and new, giving us unexpected insights and helping to forge new bonds.

We all know that those years of early parenting can take a toll on not only how you feel about yourself sexually, but on your sexual relationship with a partner. Parenting is physically demanding and there is often little energy left over for thinking about our own needs or those of our partner. When children are young tiredness is probably the crushing issue: nighttime feeding, a bedroom invaded by small bodies in the middle of the night – the incessant demands of small children can be draining on every level. I vividly remember that the only time I got to myself was when, having strapped the children into their car seats, I returned the Sainsbury's trolley to retrieve my pound! The unrelenting nature of caring for children can be doubly overwhelming for a single parent or someone without support, and the idea of considering one's own sexuality can seem laughable, while meeting someone new can feel like a logistically impossible task.

'I had a baby at 44 and found, what with the sleep deprivation and the general chaos at home, a move, elderly parents to tend to and the onset of type 1 Diabetes in my 11 month old baby, sex was not on the menu for either my husband or me. My husband also has sleep apnoea which prevents us sleeping soundly together at all times. We discussed the issue often and were not unduly stressed about it but the days turned into months and then years and we were suddenly in a marriage that resembled housemates who rear a child together... possibly a good script for an American sitcom but not what either of us planned.'
Jenny 44, Teacher

While the usual image of sex post-parenthood is the toddler sleeping peacefully between its parents, research suggests that the teenage years can impact on our sexuality just as significantly. When children are no longer tucked up safely in bed but making midnight bacon sandwiches, it can feel difficult to find privacy or space for sex, and it's difficult to give full voice to sexual passion when somebody's daubing their spots in the bathroom next door! Furthermore, when our own bodies are feeling a bit tired and saggy, it can feel as if the mantle of sexuality has been handed to these gorgeous 19-year-olds with their pert bodies and boundless stamina.

- Keep some physical affection alive even if sex has temporarily disappeared. Bedtime cuddling and kissing hello and good bye are a good start – try to do this even if you don't really feel like it.

- If you can get away for an hour, or if children are older, stimulate memories of your own teenage years and get creative about where and when. Kissing in the car or the park or just playing footsie in the pub can reintroduce a note of carefree fun.

- Go back to Way 23 and try recalling together a time or an event that inspires fond memories in you both: the first time you had sex, a time you had sex somewhere unexpected, a time when sex was utterly disastrous!

- If you have older teenagers it should be possible to leave them to their own devices and get away for a night or for a weekend. Don't however, dampen your enjoyment of time away with the weight of sexual expectation. Just focus on having some fun together away from domestic concerns. Allow anything that happens sexually to be a bonus and try not to feel that the weekend has 'failed' if you don't have sex. After all, it's said that most people don't have sex on their wedding night, surely a combination of too much alcohol and utter exhaustion but also the pressure to perform at a time when that sort of performance seems *de rigueur*!

Try taking small steps to retain some vestige of your sexual identity, just to keep a memory of it alive until it has space and time to re-emerge! Revisit the start of this book and look at Chapters 1 and 2, which focus on small ways to prioritise your independent self, rather than yourself in relation to others.

In looking after your relationship don't set your expectations too high. Try not to feel that both parties have to orgasm for sex to 'count'! It may be that full penetrative sex has to take a back seat for a while – at least until you are getting some sleep or until there's a lock on the bedroom door! In the meantime what used to be called 'heavy petting', mutual masturbation or sustained kissing can either begin to scratch a sexual itch or re-ignite a latent interest. If even that feels too demanding try putting some Chaka Khan on loud!

WAY 38 Sex in middle life

The topic of sex in middle life elicits very different responses from women. Some women welcome an end to worrying about fertility, and the menopause signals the beginning of a new sexual freedom. For others, middle life means a loss of desire and a loss of any desire *to* desire. For some women physical changes such as dryness or pain (see Ways 31 and 33) interfere with their capacity to feel sexual and sexually desiring. Sadly, I feel that at this period many women give up on feeling sexual because of the many pervasive and vastly unhelpful myths around the menopause. While the term itself simply refers to the ending of the monthly cycle, it has come to have a raft of cultural meanings around femininity, ageing and sexual attraction. However, the experience and independence that can come with middle age can allow us not only to explore sexual relationships without the encumbrances of birth control, but also to revel in our (possibly hard won) sexual self-confidence and the appeal that gives us. In order to really enjoy and explore our sexuality in middle life, we need firstly to dispel some stereotypes about who we are, what we are capable of, and what we desire in mid-life.

'I constantly need to keep my libido down. I often wonder what it would be like to talk to a man on a normal level. You go through your whole life dictated by your sexuality, eventually, as you reach middle age, you can talk to someone without that interfering.'
Eliza 48, Masseur

Reject the terminology of ageing. Undoubtedly, we live in a society that devalues older women. Terms such as *ageing gracefully* disguise attitudes to the ageing woman that are restrictive, outdated and narrow. However, the idea that middle age means being unproductive, unadventurous and physically undesirable is a stereotype that is starting to be challenged – not least because it is increasingly recognised that middle aged people are an untapped market in terms of their desire to revisit youthful 'experiences' and pursuits for example, look at the recent success of '40-plus friendly' music festivals.

Search out role models. As we did in Way 1, make a personal list of successful, intelligent and attractive women in middle age, either/ both women you know personally or those in the media spotlight. Even in the most image obsessed media such as film, middle aged actresses are increasingly being given romantic and highly sexualised film roles: Tilda Swinton, Juliette Binoche, Annette Benning, Frances McDormand, Julianne Moore among them.

Embrace your sexual appeal. By middle age you will understand your body and the scope of your sexual imagination. Drawing on your list of inspiring women (see above) remind yourself that this is a time when you can have the confidence to assert your sexuality – this is certainly not the time to hide it. Worries about our own attractiveness to others are part of our experience at any age, so accept them mindfully but put them to one side. Remember that there is nothing more sexually desirable than a confidently desiring woman. Bring to middle aged sexuality the curiosity and willingness to explore that prompted you to buy this book.

- Broaden the scope of your desires. If you are single but would like a partner it may be that your list of desirable qualities has subtly changed without you fully acknowledging how your needs have altered. Perhaps your requirements are fulfilled in some areas but not others, for example, you may enjoy living alone and want a partner who lives independently; perhaps you want to extend your interests and need a younger partner who enjoys clubbing or rock climbing.

- Middle age is a time to loosen the shackles of convention and decide what you really want and need *now* (rather than what you wanted 20 years ago or feel is appropriate for your age group).

- Try listing what you looked for in a partner in your late twenties and why (this is often a *settling down* period). Next to it list what *you* want out of your life now (think of middle age as an *up sticks* period). This might allow you to look at your needs with a fresh eye.

Don't accept temporary difficulties as inevitable: if dryness and soreness during sex is a problem, this can easily be remedied by the use of lubricants. If this continues to be a problem see your GP to discuss other options such as hormone replacement therapy. Furthermore, a sagging libido is not an inevitable consequence of reaching middle age; taking exercise, looking after your diet and actually having more sex can make you feel sexually invigorated.

WAY 39 Sex and life changes

Major changes or upheavals may interfere with both our capacity to experience ourselves as sexual individuals, and with our sex lives with a partner. For example, in middle life many of us may be coping with our children turning into adults alongside the increasing needs of elderly parents. It is as if when faced with both ends of life – the excitement of seeing our children forging their own lives independently, while our parents become frailer and more dependent – we get lost somewhere in the middle. No longer called on to care for the younger generation, we become a carer for the older. In this situation our very identity may feel nebulous and far from sexual. Change *will* happen – poor health, bereavement, break ups, redundancy – it is likely that at some point in our lives we will experience at least one, or more likely, a combination of these. In the face of major life challenges, it may be that sex and sexuality are not one of our priorities. What can we do to ensure that our sexual selves do not get entirely swallowed up by whatever trauma is threatening to engulf our sexual identity and overwhelm our sexual landscape?

'When I was threatened with redundancy, my father had recently died and at the same time I was experiencing a bout of ill health. Well, sex went straight to the bottom of the pile. In fact I felt angry at my partner for even bringing the subject up, it felt so inconsiderate. We're not out of the woods yet but what has helped a bit is making some space for myself, I do a yoga class at the weekend and I sing in a choir one evening. It does make me feel that there is something else in life for me and I've even started to feel optimistic that our love life will get back on track when things are a bit more settled.'
Fiona 52, Architect

Compartmentalise!

- If sex and sexuality have been superseded by trial and trauma, it can help to look at your life balance. Where is most of your energy going?

- The aim here is to visually represent all the elements of your life now. List all of the significant elements of your life – work, friends, relationship with partner, parenting, caring responsibilities, maintaining the home, and time spent on yourself or hobbies/things you like to do.

- Turn this into a pie chart so that you can see how much time you are devoting to each part of your life – what is the largest slice of pie? It may be that a particular section of your pie really needs your attention for the moment, but what steps can you take to increase the slice of pie dedicated to *your* needs? If all your resources are currently in the 'caring' section of your life, then your own identity, never mind the sexual side of your identity, will become submerged.

- Try to think of small things you can do to re-dress the balance. Most relationship manuals will put the focus on your relationship, but I feel strongly that this cannot be re-vitalised unless some of your energy goes into yourself – and that includes your sexual self. Go back to Chapters 1 and 2 and cherry pick, for example, nice underwear, bought by yourself for you, dancing in the kitchen while you make yourself a cocktail. Small things can increase the size of your pie slice exponentially!

- Lastly 'when laughter doesn't feature in your particular pie', be silly. When sexuality is 'sous le buffet' try stopping in the middle of one of your tedious daily routines to introduce a note of unexpected and light-hearted pleasure, either by yourself or with a partner. Do an updated Mary Poppins ('a spoonful of sugar helps the medicine go down') and give your partner an affectionate grope when you are emptying the dishwasher together. Interrupt your online banking by flipping over onto an erotic site for a few minutes, or play some Barry White on the car stereo on the way to work and sing/grunt along to the sexy bits!

40 Ageing and the sexual self

'Your sense of yourself as a sexual being changes as you get older, which can be good or bad. If you're not well, if you've got aches and pains, it does affect your feelings about your sexuality and your confidence. That's why fantasy is important.'
Joan 66, Retired

If you look up 'sexuality in older age' on Wikipedia, the very first sub heading is *Increasing Physical Limitations*. While that particular perspective is the over-riding one when it comes to sex in later life, and may well contain some truths about the difficulties experienced by some, it is time to move away from such negative stereotyping.

'I think sex gets better as you get older, you are more experienced. It gets better until it finally stops!'
Barbara 81, Retired teacher

All of us want to sustain close relationships as we grow older, and most of us feel that sex is a part of those relationships. That this should be maintained, nurtured and developed, however old we are. Many people find enormous satisfaction in sex as they grow older. Where there are no worries about pregnancy, the distractions of work and children may have lessened, and couples may have the security of a familiar partner with whom they have built up a lifelong intimacy, sex can be as good as it has ever been, or better. It seems that this once pervasive stereotype that sex comes to an end with retirement or earlier is starting to change. Highly successful movies such as *The Number One Best Exotic Marigold Hotel* show older people as adventurous and desiring, starting new lives in new places and instigating new (and sexual) relationships. Undoubtedly these new media representations of life and love in later life are only a drop in the ocean, given the many years of stereotyping around older people – but it is good news that at last there are signs of change.

'It's the same as when you were 20 because it *is* the same, but you've learned more tricks! It's better because it's not about being sexy or trying to impress someone, it's nothing to do with peacocking. It doesn't mean that you're not attractive, it comes from something deeper.'
Kate 68, Retired personnel manager

Age UK conducted an online poll, the results of which were published in 2013. This aimed to 'dispel some of the stereotypes and taboos around older people and sexual relationships'. A quarter of the older people they spoke to said that getting older has not affected their sex life and the survey showed clearly that sex remains important for people 'regardless of age'. Two thirds of those over 65s who took part said that they are currently enjoying an active and fulfilling sex life. One in eight said that they would like to try new things with a partner and about one in five said they felt they wanted to increase their sexual activity; this figure increased to over a quarter in those men polled. The main difficulty that emerged from Age UK's poll was in talking to partners and/or health professionals about sexual matters when the need arises, embarrassment being the main factor. This finding is important because sexual health remains an issue for anybody who is still sexually active and recent research has shown that, in fact, STIs (sexually transmitted infections) are on the increase amongst over 45s.

Of course sex at 60, 70 or 80 may not be quite the same as it was in your 20s but it should be possible to harness the self-assurance that comes with ageing and to feel unconstrained from those pressures to look or act a certain way that beset us when we are younger. As we age it is vital to appreciate these benefits of ageing, to value and be kind to, rather than critical of, our ageing bodies. It may be useful (at any age) to broaden our expectations and definitions of what might constitute sexual activity. If penetrative sex is difficult for any reason, take the pressure down a notch by focussing on intimacy and touch and allow other kinds of sexual act to take centre stage for a while. Having said that, there is no reason why you shouldn't maintain full intercourse if that is your desire and do seek help at any stage of life, if this is proving problematic. See Ways 31, 32 and 33.

'You can just enjoy each other. You don't have to always reach an orgasm because you know there'll always be another time to have an orgasm.'
Jean 72, Retired dentist

1 2 3 4 5 6 7 8
9 10 11 12 13 14
15 16 17 18 19
20 21 22 23 24
25 26 27 28 29
30 31 32 33 34
35 36 37 38 39
40 **41 42 43 44**
45 46 47 48 49

Chapter 9

BODY AND SOUL

Well, I said it was a journey – from Tantric sex to the cosmetics aisle (that's 'to' not 'in'). This chapter spans both the mind and the body, introducing some ways in which mindful meditation can unlock the potential of our sexuality, and how yoga may be used as a way of releasing sexual energy in the body. We also look at issues around body confidence and the significance of posture.

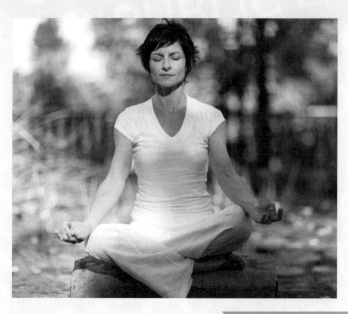

My body, a cause of joy

Much has been written in recent years, both in the popular and in the academic press, about the 'pornification' or sexualisation of our culture. This idea refers to the increasing mainstreaming of sexuality, and encompasses a huge range of things, from pole dancing kits for sale in Tesco to late night television programmes on how to have better sex with your partner. A book such as this one, for sale in a mainstream book shop and perhaps read openly on the tube or on the bus, could be said to be part of the 'sexualisation' of our culture. The move towards greater visibility in sexual matters, including an emphasis on performance, technique and sexual gratification has inevitably changed the way that we think about and experience our sexuality. Some will proclaim this as a good thing, a sign of an increased openness in society, in which marginalised groups, women, gay men and lesbians, can discuss their needs openly and without censure. On the other hand, for some people the unambiguously sexual imagery with which we are bombarded daily diminishes our understanding of sexuality as something both deeply personal and transcendent.

Clearly, in many cultures and for many religious persuasions sexuality has a profound importance that may be linked to marriage and the family. While many of us do not participate in organised religion, it may be that the 'commodification' of our sexuality leaves little room for feelings that the sexual act is a private, profound and even spiritual connection with another person. Rowan Williams, former Archbishop of Canterbury said in a lecture in 1989:

'For my body to be the cause of joy, the end of homecoming, for me, it must be there for someone else, be perceived, accepted, nurtured; and that means being given over to the creation of joy in that other... To desire my joy is to desire the joy of the one I desire: my search for enjoyment through the bodily presence of another is a longing to be enjoyed in my body.'

If we are to see sex as a vehicle for joy in ourselves and others, then cherishing and revering our own sexual identity is not merely a matter of wearing nice underwear and lighting some scented candles, but an act which nurtures us at the deepest level in order that we can celebrate sexuality in all its manifestations. For many people, practices originating in Eastern religions and cultures have been one route to re-establishing sexuality as a manifestation of the spiritual. Many cultures have celebrated sexual ecstasy as a means to the divine, the most well-known being Tantric sex, in reality a Western practice which has loosely appropriated Taoist and Buddist tantra principles. Some meditation practices have much in common with the precepts of Indian yoga, the idea of energy channels within the body linking chakras or energy points.

This is an exercise based on the principles of Akashic meditation:

An expert in this form of meditation is said to be rewarded with intense experiences through which they can understand the sexual desires of all people, the experiences of the entire animal kingdom, and truly understand the limitless potential of their own lust!

Step one Every day we are told what to do and what not to do, we are given specific instructions on what is possible. But, for this moment, you must accept that these rules are paper thin and liable to blow away with the slightest wind.

Step two Begin your meditation by closing your eyes and relinquishing your fear. Your fear stems from the idea of loss, the idea that you exist in a world where loss can be forced upon you, and because of this, we often try to protect ourselves. We must accept our fragility and embrace it, for it is the fragility we all share and there is nothing wrong with acknowledging vulnerability.

Step three Sit cross legged with your bottom firmly planted on the floor (if this is difficult, sit on a chair). Ensure that you're comfortable in this position and slowly breathe in and out five times, visualising the negative energy as it leaves with the exhalation, and the positive energy as it enters with the inhalation.

Step four Ground your body by ensuring that your spine is straight and that you are anchored, by placing one or both hands in front of you as you feel the need.

Step five As we move closer you must forget your surroundings as they are unimportant to your meditation, and embrace the animal side of your sexuality. As you breathe you must visualise who you are, the person who accepts their sexuality without apology or consequence.

WAY 42 — Yoga and the sexual you

While Way 41 focused on visualisation and the mind, Ways 42 and 43 begin to unite mind and body through yoga practice. Yoga has been used for centuries as a way of connecting mind, body and spirit to harness a healing sexual energy. Below, one of my research participants explains how yoga has had practical benefits both for herself and for her sex life with her partner.

'I have practised yoga on and off for many years and have always found my way back to health and happiness via the assanas and some meditation. I am not a natural meditator and my husband was new to yoga, but we found regular practice of Astanga and some monthly Kundalini classes really boosted our flagging libidos and gave us something to talk about other than blood glucose levels and the car insurance. Kundalini is particularly useful in boosting libido as the practice focuses somewhat on the base of the spine – the 'kundalini' is imagined as a spiral which when activated by good practise energises and opens the chakras above this area, creating harmony, both physical and spiritual. It is not uncommon for a Kundalini yoga practitioner to warn students of the possible libido uplift, yes, erections in class and a spring in the step, skip lunch and rush home for some action... Hilarious, but we found it really worked and we are much more relaxed about everything in general, which helps. We had both become quite anxious about sex with each other and even admitted to very infrequent masturbation. Yoga saved the day and whilst we are hardly blushing newly-weds, we do occasionally have to lock the bedroom door!'

Gabriella 45, Dental technician

Yoga has been found to be beneficial in increasing flexibility, body strength and reducing stress levels, all important factors when working on revitalizing or invigorating our sexuality. However, traditionally it has also been used to harness and channel sexual energy to increase physical health, develop individual well-being and improve our sex lives.

Emma Cole, yoga teacher, offers a yoga position that she uses in her own teaching for releasing and enhancing sexual energy and explains the thinking behind it:

Sexual expression/sexuality is the domain of the 2nd chakra in yoga, also called 'svadisthana chakra' meaning 'one's own abode'. This is located in the pelvic area and is associated with the water element – it is liquid, moist, fluid. The following exercises focus on the hips, the sacrum, the lower abdomen and the pelvis. In order to reach a state of 'flow' it is important to do all these exercises from a relaxed place, so some time needs to be spent relaxing before you start.

1. Pelvic rock/sacral massage

Lying on the back with knees bent – take at least five breaths there to allow the body to settle, with a focus on releasing the back of the sacrum into the floor – letting it completely relax, feel the structure of the pelvis and visualize it with your mind's eye. Also let the back settle properly, so shoulders are relaxed and the landscape of the back relaxes completely. Use mindful breathing as a focus for relaxing: sense and feel both the in-breath and the out-breath. Notice what happens to the body whilst breathing, the rise and fall of the chest, the temperature of the breath. Relax key areas like the jaw and soften the skin of the face (in somatic practices there is a lot of research being done on the connection between the jaw and the pelvis!).

Then, feeling the pelvis as very heavy, begin to gently tilt the pelvis forwards and tuck it back under, like you're giving your sacrum a massage. Enjoy the feeling of the sacrum being massaged by the movement against the ground, explore the ability to feel pleasure and give yourself permission to enjoy this simple massage.

Here we are awakening the kundalini energy with sensual stimulation. After a couple of minutes just release the movement and become still, relax and observe any feelings in the pelvis, sacrum, hips etc. Just be present to sensation.

WAY 43 Energy, strength, sensation

One of the major benefits of yoga is the way in which it teaches us to trust in and be aware of our bodies, to pay attention to our posture and to maintain this focus even in daily life. The following yoga poses, also from Emma Cole, focus on our pelvic floor area, genitals and finally and joyfully, some therapeutic bottom wobbling!

2. Moola bhanda with kumbhaka

'Bhandas' (energetic seals/locks) are a well-known concept in yoga and are used all the time. There are three main ones but this one corresponds to the 2nd chakra.

This one means 'root lock' or 'root seal', and is also known as 'the master key' in yoga. I find this incredibly potent as it exercises the pelvic floor and the cervical contraction is much like the contraction one has during orgasm. It stimulates the muscles and nerves of the pelvic region and so builds energy, strength, sensation and awareness there, all of which arouse the area.

It's basically the same thing as a 'pelvic floor exercise' – but with extra breath focus, squeezing the pelvic floor in and up and releasing it. It's great to do this at the end of an in-breath, then don't breathe out for about 4/6/8 seconds (this is called kumbakha/breath retention), then release the breath and the bandha.

3. Still poses

Malasana/Garland Pose A deep squat which opens up the 1st/root chakra and gets into the hips. Here we can begin to connect down into the earth and stimulate the hips, opening the genital area!

Supta Tarasana/Reclined Goddess (a great pose for a meditation) Lie on your back, knees bent a little way in, then drop the knees out to the side and bring the soles of the feet together. Rest the hands softly on the lower abdomen. Breathe.

Try to let the hips completely relax and gently work with the breath until the hip flexors release and the legs fall open naturally, and the thighs and buttocks aren't gripping. If you're really tight in the hips you can use rolled up towels/pillows underneath each thigh so the legs can rest and be supported on them. Then you unfold energetically. You can use visualisation here, for example, a rose flowering in the lower abdomen. Try visualising its colour, scent and so on, see the petals unfolding in your mind's eye. Stay for 3–5 minutes. Try using music and smells that evoke sensuality to enhance the pose.

4. Standing pose

Heel pummeling

Stand with feet hip width apart, toes forward, knees soft (i.e. have a slight bend in the knees). Feel the soles of the feet melt into the ground, close your eyes, breathe, feel.

Begin to pummel the heels alternately, lifting and 'plonking' them down, fast and vigorously so that it becomes like a drum-roll! As long as the knees are bent then this is easy – if you lock the knees it becomes really awkward. I always encourage my students to jiggle and wobble and let their bum flesh wobble as much as possible and it always makes them laugh with joy! It's so freeing and liberating to let the flesh of the bottom be wobbled and shaken up.

44 A word on body confidence

Emma's heel pummelling exercise in Way 43 is a great way to introduce a section on *body confidence* and to enjoy the sensation of our moving bodies, increasing our understanding of what bodies can do!

Body confidence inevitably plays a highly significant part in how we feel about ourselves, whether we see ourselves as sexual women and whether we allow ourselves to be attracted to and attractive to others. We all know perfectly well that the images of 'flawless femininity' with which we are bombarded daily via a variety of media, are highly manipulated images of women in their late teens and early 20s. Nevertheless, this perpetual onslaught of a very narrowly defined version of perfection is liable to erode any shred of body confidence we have managed to dredge up from somewhere. Personally, I struggle with summer – the prospect of emerging white and dimpled from my happy cocoon of woolly jumpers and black tights is less than appealing. I tend to search the online BBC weather with mounting anxiety, only relieved when I triumphantly encounter the familiar icon of a black cloud with a single raindrop poised to fall from its bottom.

Bodies are about how we feel, rather than how we are, and so our body confidence is based on how we feel about ourselves, rather than on fact or on empirically-based evidence. Because body confidence is so entirely subjective, it changes from day to day and is very easily influenced and distorted by external factors which we internalise in the form of self-doubt, self-criticism and even self-loathing. Holding up those media images of unblemished adolescent 'perfection' as an ideal to which we should aspire means that we are in a constant battle with our body. Inevitably, we know that this is a battle we are destined to lose – or brands and advertisers wouldn't reap the huge rewards of our dissatisfaction.

This dispiriting and disempowering state of affairs can also impact on our motivation to look after our bodies, for example, not going swimming owing to a fear of revealing what we think of as a less than perfect body. A healthy body image is one that allows us to be comfortable with what we have, to recognise its strengths and accept 'imperfections' as common to everybody. A healthy body image allows us to really enjoy and nurture our bodies. Cognitive behavioural therapy techniques can be really useful in helping us to look clearly and realistically at our physical appearance (see *49 Ways to Think Yourself Well* for useful exercises to help you break the cycle of negative comparison and see and experience your body more positively).

Last year I was on a beach in Italy. Italy has always seemed to me a place where appearance is paramount to all, but on that beach were women of all ages from 18 to 75 or more and they were *all*, every one of them, in bikinis. I don't think those women were wearing bikinis to look sexy, not one of them was sucking in her stomach or carefully arranging her limbs to look more streamlined. Those women were enjoying the sun (harmful exposure to UV rays is another topic entirely!) on as much of their bodies as possible, and wallowing in the sensation of the water on their skin. For me that beach was something of an epiphany!

I'll be doing this one too, and it works well in a group:

- Firstly, ask everybody to draw a picture of themselves. You can make these simple or more elaborate but it doesn't matter tuppence how bad at drawing you are.

- Using arrows to point to the drawing, everyone should list at least five things they like about their body and/or face. The more the better.

- Then they can point to one thing they don't like, but *only* one! This could be in another colour.

- Take it in turns to hold up your picture and explain what that you like about your body in some detail. Give reasons: 'I like my thighs because I do a lot of cycling, it's something I really enjoy and it has made me fit.'

Of course, you can do this exercise alone but it works best as a way of breaking that cycle of mutual body dissatisfaction and negative one-upmanship that women often indulge in, for example, 'I hate my arms' … 'You hate *your* arms, yours are fine, you should see *my* arms', and so on! The aim of this exercise is to take a step towards breaking down the very narrow framework within which we judge ourselves and to encourage women to celebrate their bodies on a far broader basis. Plus it's important to hear other women's reasons for celebrating their own bodies.

WAY 45 On deportment

At the start of this book I suggested that this book represents a journey we will go on together. Well, as I write this chapter I have a back and neck problem that, in addition to causing me quite a lot of pain, has prompted me to think in a way I never have before about the relationship between my own body and how I feel about myself sexually. I have found it difficult to feel good about myself – in any way, let alone sexually – now my body is in revolt, now that I am limited in what I can do. I am only too conscious that my formerly ramrod straight back is now (in my mind anyway!) contorted and bent. Like all of us, I have taken my body largely for granted until, for whatever reason, it is not working properly, so if you'll allow me, I want to share a few thoughts with you gleaned from my own recent experience.

Our bodies speak. Our posture is a reflection of how we feel about ourselves; our posture gives the world a clear message about our self-confidence and self-esteem, our health and well-being, and speaks volumes about how we view ourselves sexually. As a lecturer, I have often coached students in how to give effective presentations. We are all well accustomed to the idea that our body language is a large component of how others view us in the context of performance, interview and so on. Since my own body has turned against me, I'm all too aware that the signals it is sending to others are also reverberating in my own mind: 'I'm broken, I'm slow, I'm ageing, I can't do things'. All in all, I'm increasingly realising how much of my self-esteem, (including, or particularly, sexual self-esteem) resides in my posture and my ability to move freely and easily.

As we all increasingly spend long periods at a computer, our posture tends to sink, our shoulders fall forwards, often our upper backs weaken, and we appear to lose height. Here I want you to spend some time thinking around how you might experiment with the impact your posture has on how you feel about yourself.

I tried this while shopping in Boots and was truly astonished – it is such a simple thing but for a brief moment I think I occupied a slightly larger space in the cosmetics aisle!

- Chose a social interaction that involves you speaking to someone unfamiliar. This can simply be buying something in a shop, taking something to the dry cleaners, speaking to a new neighbour. It doesn't have to be someone of the opposite sex, this is about your self-perception not attracting a potential partner.

- Without looking utterly ridiculous as you chat to the dry cleaner about the unseemly stains on your little black dress, allow your shoulders to move forwards and down – the aim is that during the exchange you should adopt a slightly more exaggerated, tired, slumped posture than is usual to you.

- Now you know what I'm going to say! Take another similar situation and do the opposite. As you buy your weekly lottery ticket, pint of milk, compensatory bar of Cadbury's, stand straight (try placing one hand on your tummy about the height of an imaginary belt buckle and press in slightly), relax your shoulders, drop your chin (push it down and backwards slightly with the fingers of your other hand to help align your neck) and notice the difference in how you feel about yourself. You might be having a giggle with the shop assistant by this point if nothing else!

Improved posture obviously means less back and neck problems, but it also impacts on our interactions with the world. It is a little like that old idea of 'fake it to make it'. An erect body posture ensures that others see you as confident in your own skin, and projecting self-assurance is a big step towards actually acquiring it. Let's briefly go back to Rowan Williams:

'For my body to be the cause of joy, the end of homecoming, for me, it must be there for someone else, be perceived, accepted, nurtured.'

Just now I need to accept and nurture this complaining body of mine. I cannot say that it is currently a cause of joy, but for one brief moment in Boots it was getting there and that was largely because of my recognition of how I was *perceived* when I adjusted my *posture*.

References

Anodea, J. (2004) *Eastern Body, Western Mind*. Celestial Arts.

Alcoe, J., Gajewski, E. (2013) *49 Ways to Think Yourself Well*, Brighton: Step Beach Press.

1 2 3 4 5 6 7 8
9 10 11 12 13 14
15 16 17 18 19
20 21 22 23 24
25 26 27 28 29
30 31 32 33 34
35 36 37 38 39
40 41 42 43 44
45 **46 47 48 49**

Chapter 10

IN IT FOR THE LONG HAUL

The one sexual relationship we are certainly in for the long haul is the one we have with ourselves. This chapter looks back at how we might move forward in our journey to sexual self-actualisation, and also at what might prevent us from fully exploring our sexual nature. It examines the ways in which a 'mindful' approach to looking at the 'now' might help us to be accepting and non-judgemental of ourselves, and lastly offers a quick, light-hearted and personal recap as we part company.

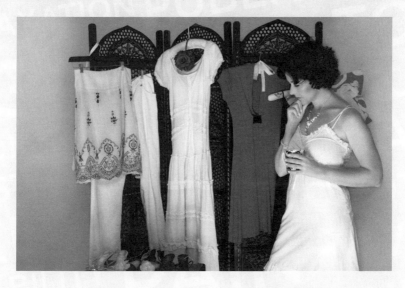

46 The newly sexual you: public not private

When we make changes in our lives it is our nature to crave feedback in order to validate those changes, we need them to be noticed, to be reflected back to us. A previously large friend of mine has recently lost a huge amount of weight: she tells me that she cannot see it and only really believes it when she encounters the surprise and congratulations of others.

We have been talking about making subtle changes in ourselves, in our attitudes, in our openness to new things, in order to fully embrace our sexuality. Like my friend, we will need this to be noticed and celebrated by the people around us, we will need to see some corresponding change in the way that others respond to us. In other words, we will need evidence that what we are doing is making some change in our lives. But this is complicated, isn't it, when it comes to sexuality – surely sex is a very private matter and not for public consumption?

Think about what you can do to turn your private acknowledgement of the place of sexuality in your world, into a public statement. 'Oh no' I hear you say, 'What are you suggesting?'. Think back over what you have read so far. What small concrete changes can you make now?

Early on in this book we started to identify what sexuality means for us by thinking about personal role models. Doing the following exercise will help you to reinforce this, allowing you to identify what it is that might *signal* the you who has embraced her sexuality, the you who is comfortable and secure in her sexual nature.

This is a visualisation exercise:

- Start by finding somewhere quiet and doing some deep breathing exercises to relax your mind. Notice sounds and sensation, but they are simply that – try to let them drift past you.

- Picture yourself as if you were watching the new you on a cinema screen. Start to imagine the new, sexually self-actualised you.

- What are you doing? What are you wearing? How are you standing/sitting?

- Now make the picture even more vivid. Add some detail to the image. Where are you? What is the weather like? Who is around you or who are you with? Can you hear any sounds. What are they?

- Then make the screen larger, and the colours brighter, try to hear the sounds and then amplify them. (You have gone IMAX!)

- Lastly, imagine yourself walking into the huge image of yourself on the screen (in a Sci Fi, Star Trek sort of way!) Walk into yourself and fully inhabit that image. Continue to experience the sounds, smells and colours around you for a few moments.

For further guidance on using the power of visualisation see *49 Ways to Think Yourself Well*.

We discussed the idea of a 'sexy' woman (see Way 1) and discounted the stereotypical media image of what she looks like. This exercise is designed to help you to define what 'embracing your sexuality' actually *looks like* – and for you specifically.

It may help at this point to make a few brief notes: what did you focus on, was it your posture, your clothes, the colours you were wearing, the language you were using or how you were speaking, for example? Finally, spend some time thinking about how you might begin to move towards this sexually confident you. What small changes could you make now that will signal to others that you are a woman who is comfortable with your sexual self?

Sometimes, doing something unexpected can prompt others to see you in a new way and be a trigger for a more profound alteration in your view of yourself. It can be something very small and seemingly insignificant.

WAY 47 Barriers to becoming the new sexual you

Now you have formed a strong visual image of the newly sexually self-confident and comfortable you, it is worth spending some time thinking about what small steps you might take to get closer to being that person you saw on your internal cinema screen. It may also be helpful at this point to take a moment to examine what factors or unhelpful core beliefs might get in the way of your achieving this.

For example, we have discussed various forms of stereotype including the 'sexy' woman, the perfect body, stereotypical thinking around sexuality and the older woman. We have begun to think about how these limited, narrow and unenlightened patterns of representing women might impact on our understanding and beliefs about what it means to be a sexual woman.

In a very personal sense we may find that we have internalised these widespread cultural beliefs around female sexuality. These deeply entrenched ways of thinking may form a barrier which prevent us from fully enjoying and inhabiting our sexuality – we are too fat, too thin, too old, too married, too single, too busy to be the woman who is able to explore and express her sexual identity with confidence and an open mind. What's more it is difficult to let go of these beliefs because at some level we experience our fears and inhibitions as the very things that are protecting us from danger, from the censure or ridicule of those around us. Do we feel that if we start to experiment with our appearance, we may end up looking ridiculous? Are we frightened that if we visit a sex shop somebody may see us going in and judge us? Are we scared that if we begin to explore our sexuality and our sexual feelings we will lose control? Do we believe we have to dampen our sexual feelings as we exit the menopause?

In this book we have challenged many of these negative stereotypes; for example, we have rejected the terminology of ageing, banned the idea of being age appropriate in dress or behaviour, and embraced fantasy and visual stimulation. We have used visualisation, meditation and yoga to prompt us to look at ourselves in relation to healthy positive role models, to release sexual energy and to help us take a positive approach to sexuality and any sexual difficulties we encounter. Finally, in order to put up a strong challenge to those things which prevent us embracing our sexuality, we must identify just what we gain from clinging to these very disobliging and unhelpful beliefs. In other words – we have to move the sideboard!

Can you identify the fears you may need to overcome in order to fully embrace your sexuality? Can you start to look at what those fears and barriers might be protecting you from?

Try drawing yourself three columns. In the first column write down the fear. Then think what it is protecting you from – this could be one thing or many things. Lastly, use a third column to start challenging the validity of those beliefs. For example:

The fear	is protecting me from	But
I am nervous about using erotic material on the internet to stimulate myself.	People thinking badly of me. Seeing something I don't want to see. Not being a good feminist, demeaning myself and other women. No longer finding my partner arousing.	This is just for me, nobody else needs to know. If I don't like it I can move on and delete it from my browsing history. I can look at a woman friendly site, made by women for women. Erotic material may stimulate my fantasies and bring something new to love making.

Finally, look back at what it was that made you pick up this book in the first place and what you hoped it might offer you. Can you identify any pre-conceptions around sexuality which you brought to reading this book? In what ways do you think these pre-conceptions have been tested or refuted in the course of reading this book?

WAY 48 Knowing me by now

Mindfulness is a very current concept which stems from meditative practice, itself originating in Buddhism. It is now being used extensively as a way of alleviating a variety of mental and physical conditions such as pain, anxiety and depression. In essence, it is a way attempting to bring one's full attention to present experience. Mindfulness involves an awareness of sensations and thoughts as they inevitably travel through the mind, an awareness which is entirely non-judgemental – which maintains openness and acceptance.

However, I find the word 'mindfulness' something of a contradiction in terms of a practice that offers to still the mind by inhabiting the moment. I prefer the term 'nowness' which for me embodies this idea of being fully present, while not *engaging* with the meanderings of our restless brains. Clearly this idea of 'nowness' has resonances when we are considering our experience of sexuality, its focus on being accepting and non-judgemental is particularly relevant here since we all inevitably bring to sexuality so much baggage in terms of past experience, feelings of guilt, self-recrimination and so on. Mindful sexuality a ttempts to focus purely on sensation, on the feeling of one's skin against taut sheets, the smell of a lover's hair, the body's response to stimulation, allowing us to experience sex, free from the inhibition prompted by an ever vigilant mind.

However, while this practice can be invaluable in helping us to fully inhabit the act of sex, either alone or with a partner, don't reserve the idea of 'nowness' solely for those moments of 'doing' sex. Practising 'nowness' in the everyday will certainly help us to still our minds, allowing us to prioritise our sensuous response to the world we inhabit. One of the most important spiritual teachings to have emerged from the 21st century is this idea that all your experiences should be seen and understood in the very moment they exist. There is nothing more intense than properly experienced sexual urges and the key to achieving your sexual awakening may lie with this concept of nowness.

First, we must accept that the future is unknown. We like to feel that we can predict the future and, when most of us try this, we use our past to form our expectations. We must abandon our expectations. It is hard to live a full life without experiencing negative events, but we must leave our negative emotions behind, that perhaps stemmed from times when we were not at our most sexual or when we were made to feel guilty about our natural sexual energies. To fully accept an open future you must fully accept the immaterial nature of the past.

We can use anything we want to inform our futures, so to reach our peak of sexual inhibition we must bring our most sexual persona out of our imagination.

Second, we must accept that the past is unknown. We may have been made to feel bad about our past experiences; whilst we can remember a narrative of the past, we must not judge these events, and as time passes we must not continue to react to events we no longer experience.

Conflict between sexual energies and our emotions is a very common experience and it is important to accept both independently and not to judge either. Understand that they are both a part of you, and that they can exist in duality without compromising each other. Shame is another important emotion to abandon when in the moment. We are all sexual creatures and no-one is fit to judge us in any way for simply being sexual. Being sexual is the most natural thing in the world.

To fully embrace the nowness of your experience you must practise. This can be done whilst alone or with a partner, and can be done with new experiences or with old ones:

- Try new things, perhaps slowly at first. Return to Way 2, which stresses the importance of spending time alone but with others. Practise focusing on bodily sensation as you do this, for example, the weight of your bottom on a café chair, the resistance of water as you swim.
- Try familiar things as if they were new experiences, for example, as you undertake an everyday or mundane task such as cooking a meal or having a shower, focus on physical sensation, notice your thoughts as if they are passing before you on a cinema screen.
- Concentrate on and notice what you feel, rather than what you are supposed to feel. It is very difficult to disentangle the two but a powerfully enlightening exercise to attempt.
- Don't compare yourself physically against someone who doesn't exist. Recall Way 44 and know that your body is simply curves and lines.
- Immerse yourself in your physical response to erotic stimuli. Acknowledge and accept, but try not to engage with, any self-monitoring or self-criticism which passes through your mind as you do this.
- Remember sexual experience and sexual feelings are neither negative nor positive.

WAY 49

Out from underneath the sideboard!

I said at the start that this book would be a road we travel together. Now, as I am writing this, I am attempting to picture you as you rifle through your underwear drawer, sit up ramrod straight and flirt with the barrista in Caffé Nero, I wish we could share a giggle together! Rather than re-capping in any formal sense I want to share with you what has resonated for me over the process of writing and researching this book.

These are the things that stand out for me if we are to retrieve our sexuality from underneath that sideboard. First of all sexuality does, and it should pervade our everyday lives. The notion that we are sexual beings comes easily to us when we are young, indeed the media would have us believe that sexuality is the province of the young. As we live lives increasingly full of responsibility and restraint, our sense of ourselves as sexual beings in the world may be mislaid, lost or buried, either through our own carelessness, as a response to societal pressures, or because it has sunk to the bottom of a growing pile of things to attend to. .

Sometimes I find myself foraging to retrieve a sense of my own Sexuality. A sexual self that I seem to recall I left somewhere under a huge mound of other, seemingly more important, things. I suggest that you imagine yourself burrowing away at that pile, tossing aside those aspects of your life that suppress or hinder expression of the sexual you, including both the dowdy shoes and that dampening sense of what is inappropriate – that inhibiting habit of self-monitoring. Start by finding your own visual image, one that works for you in encapsulating this ongoing process of discarding, retrieving and unearthing and return to it daily.

Make room for frisson. Collect and practise a few flirting techniques and allow everyday encounters to venture ever so slightly outside the confines of the conventional. Gentle flirting with my very nice middle aged, Turkish dry cleaner has led to fascinating conversations about current events, an invitation to his villa in Cyprus, not to mention extra speedy dry cleaning! The sense that somebody is looking at you with interest, not born out of your capacity to help them with their homework but because you appear attractive, interesting and fun – is a highly efficient way of reminding yourself that you are or have the capacity to be, that person.

Clothes are a source of fun and, importantly, have a significant impact on how you feel about your sexual persona. Personally, I have bought better knickers for everyday wear. Black hipster knickers, they are functional, fit well under clothes but are not knickers to be ashamed of. On the other hand, allow yourself to experiment joyfully with clothes, banish the 'I can't possibly wear that' mantra. Be Italian:; buy a bikini, not simply because it may look sexy on the beach at Bridlington but because you will revel in the sensation of the sun (if you're lucky) on your skin. Re-invent your personal aesthetic, whether you want to play with classic neutrals, sculptural shapes and red lipstick or investigate colour, pattern or vintage styles – give yourself permission to try out new identities, new modes of being yourself.

Fantasy is paramount, without fantasy there is no arousal – but we have banished a narrow understanding of both these terms. Don't save fantasy for the bedroom, let it into your everyday life. Release any prejudice you may have about visual or written erotica and dip a toe into the water if you haven't already. Finally, return to the visualisation exercises in Chapter 1, incorporate ideas of 'nowness' from Way 48 and allow yourself to exercise your sexual self in surprising contexts.

Don't underestimate the power and importance of the physical in helping you to *let in* a sense of your own sexual nature – to revitalize, rejuvenate and empower you. Dance, sing, practise the yoga exercises from Ways 42 and 43 to release and harness a sexual energy which may have been diminished or suppressed by the unremitting demands of dailyness.

This is vital. Make time in your day or week, to be alone in a crowd. Remember, this is not time to make to-do lists, send texts or call your mother/daughter/ best friend who needs your attention. This is a time to allow your imagination to wander, to fantasise and, importantly, to allow yourself to receive gracefully and unresistingly any curiosity you sense others may have about you. Try using the idea of 'nowness' in this context.

If you take one thing away with you from this book it should be that sexuality starts with you as an independent individual, not you in relation to others. In order to bring your sexuality to a relationship, you must first explore, nurture and ultimately revel in, your own sexual self.

FURTHER INFORMATION, READING AND RESOURCES

Chapter 1

Way 5 Doing sexuality

Play list

- Serge Gainsbourg – *Je T'Aime Moi Non Plus*
- Barry White – *Never Gonna Give You Up*
- The Doors – *Love Her Madly*
- Alicia Keys – *Harlem's Nocturne*
- Joan Armatrading – *The Weakness In Me*
- Nelly – *Hot In Here*
- Sidney Bechet – *I Only Have Eyes for You*
- Marvin Gaye – *Sexual Healing*
- Nina Simone – *I Want a Little Sugar in My Bowl*
- Marvin Gaye – *Let's Get It On*
- Donna Summer – *I Feel Love*
- Barry White – *Can't Get Enough of Your Love, Babe*
- Van Morrison – *TB Sheets*
- Otis Redding – *Try a Little Tenderness*
- Touch & To – *Would You*
- Barbra Streisand – *Evergreen* (love theme for *A Star is Born*)

Chapter 3

Way 15 Sex in cyberspace

Blogs:

- www.tinynibbles.com A blog by American writer Violet Blue, award-winning sex author and columnist, as well as an expert in the field of sex and technology. Much more than a sex blog, her work is both informative and discursive covering a wide range of current issues under the loose umbrella of sexuality – well worth a look.

- popmycherryreview.com An American sex toy review blog run by Domina Doll featuring reviews of American sex toys, many of which are also available online from British stores. It includes sex toy reviews and advice as well as adult film and movie reviews with a focus on porn for women. Who knew you could buy a lockable vibrator case?

- boobaloosreviews.com/about-me/ A blog that reviews sex toys from a independent and personal perspective.

Discussion platforms and review and information sites:

- ourpornourselves.org/ Our Porn Ourselves is a resource that aims to create an alternative and constructive conversation on the use of pornography by women, and in turn offer balance to the anti-porn feminist agenda.

- www.sexuality.org/ A pioneering American site no longer actively maintained, it is still a useful resource. It has useful reviews and links to books and films for women as well as information on a wide variety of sexual practices.

- eroticaforall.co.uk/about/ A site for readers and writers of erotica.

- www.thefword.org.uk/ A discussion platform for contemporary UK feminism.

- clitical.com A site that celebrates female self-pleasure and contains erotic stories, sex toy reviews and so on.

Women focused porn, made by women, for women:

The following are women film makers of erotic films:

Anna Span makes movies, some of which are R18s and which can only be sold on licensed premises, and some are 18s, which means that you can choose how explicit you would like your movie to be.

- Anna Span
- Petra Joy
- Candida Royalle
- xconfessions.com/erika-lust/Erika Lust. Lust is an independent erotic filmmaker, author, and founder of Erika Lust Films. Lust aims to show the feminine viewpoint in erotica.
- See www.pornmoviesforwomen.com/femaleporndirectors.htm for a comprehensive list of female directors of erotic movies.

Chapter 4
Way 16 The stereotype of sex shopping: don't let it get in the way of a fun day out!

The following shops pride themselves on being woman friendly. All these shops offer a safe, comfortable experience for shoppers where they can browse at their leisure and where help and advice is available should they need it.

- **Sh!** Branches in London's Hoxton and Notting Hill. Sh! is the first sex shop set up in the early 1990s to cater solely to the needs of women, highly inclusive in all respects, it caters to both straight and gay women. All their products are tested by the team and while the atmosphere is light-hearted, novelty for novelty's sake is discouraged, as is packaging featuring pouting pneumatic blondes. Sh! is a very welcoming space which only lets men into the shop if they are accompanied by a woman, staff are friendly, knowledgeable and utterly un-judgemental. Sh! is an excellent place to buy your first sex toy,

there is a display in the shop where you can try out the vibrating toys and while you will not be pressured, down to earth advice will be available should you need it.

Sh! also has a good, if slightly busy, website which features not only a wide range of products but useful advice and feedback from consumers.

- **Ann Summers** will be familiar to everybody – on every high street it has responded to the new market for woman-friendly sexual products by improving the look of their shops as well as their underwear. While it does retain a jokey, hen party ambiance, it is an accessible and unthreatening shop to enter.
- **Coco de Mer** is a luxurious and exclusive female-friendly sex shop in London's Covent Garden. It sells a range of the more expensive and even designer sex toys and acoutrements, as well as beautiful lingerie and books. Coco de Mer also holds 'salons' where you can learn the art of spanking or to play the 'flute' as well as other slightly esoteric pleasures. Good for a mooch around even if you don't buy anything – don't be intimidated by its upmarket atmosphere.

Coco de Mer also has a stylish website which sometimes features a promotional video made by a well known director displaying the attractions of the current face of Coco de Mer; at one time Kate Moss or Maggie Gyllenhaal.

- **She Said**, Ship Street, Brighton. A friendly and somewhat upmarket shop in Brighton which has a carefully chosen product range as well as beautiful lingerie, burlesque wear and costumes. It offers a very pleasant and attractive shopping experience and the well informed service that you will find in many of the women-friendly stores. She Said has a good website (www.shesaidboutique.com) which is not overwhelming.

Women-friendly retail websites

- www.sh-womenstore.com Sh! has a carefully selected but wide range of toys and books etc. It also features useful user reviews as well as advice on what to buy for your needs and sex advice. A slightly overly informative site in terms of design but a company I recommend heartily for their genuine interest in their female clientele and inclusive attitude to sexuality.

- www.annsummers.com has a wide range of sex toys: you will need to be selective.

- coco-de-mer.com has exclusive toys, upmarket bondage accessories and lingerie.

- www.love honey.com

- www.whistleandhum.co.uk

- www.babes-n-horny.com for dildos and harnesses in fabulous colours and designs.

- www.beecourse.com A women and couples-friendly site which, like many female-friendly sex shops, prides itself on customer service. It has an informative website with useful tips and advice on rather more than sex toys.

Chapter 5

Way 25 Discussing your sexuality with a professional

How to find a sex therapist:

Unfortunately, current NHS policy, alongside cuts in funding, mean that approaching your GP for sex therapy is unlikely to guarantee help on the NHS although he or she may well be able to point you in the direction of private support. Here are some useful starting points for which you do not need a GP referral:

- **Relate** provides sex therapy for couples and individuals. Contact Relate directly for therapists local to you, they also offer live chat sessions with a trained relate counsellor. See relate.org.uk

- **The College of Sexual and Relationship Therapists** COSRT is a membership organization for all therapists specialising in sexual and relationship issues, it is a major provider of professional support to members and is a training provider. Their website offers a directory of all COSRT members at cosrt.org.uk. Fees will vary between therapists and different parts of the country.

Chapter 7

Way 34 Sex and Mental Health: depression and SSRIs
Way 35: Sex and disability

Further reading:

The Ultimate Guide To Sex and Disability by Mirium Kaugman, Cory Silverberg and Fran Odette, published by Cleis Press in 2003 but updated in 2007. This is a very useful and comprehensive guide that covers a huge range of disabilities, from chronic fatigue syndrome to spinal cord injury. It promises to give you 'everything you need to know to create a sex life that works for you', including sexual positions to minimise stress and maximise pleasure and building a positive sexual self-image. It is recommended for its huge scope and accessible style.

Shopping:

For some people particular sex toys may be helpful. You may have realized by now that I am a bit of a fan of this shop, however if you would like to experiment with sex toys, I recommend contacting www.sh-womenstore.com who have worked with health services and are well informed and helpful. They will offer advice if you need something that will meet specific needs.

Useful websites:

- www.sexualityanddisability.org
  Sexuality and Disability is 'a website that starts with the premise that women who are disabled are sexual beings – just like any other woman'. The site frankly and informatively covers a wide range of topics around sexuality. It confronts the questions that may be asked by any woman with a disability: questions around the 'mechanics' of having sex, being in a relationship, fears around abuse, experience of having children and so on.

- www.tlc-trust.org.uk The TLC Trust was founded in 2000 at a Sexual Freedom Coalition Conference, entitled *Let's Start the Real Sexual Revolution.* One of the speakers, James Palmer, a disabled man, revealed his sadness at being a virgin in his mid 40s. Through its excellent, accessible and comprehensive website, the TLC Trust website provides opportunities, advice and support to men and women with a huge range of disabilities so they can find appropriate sexual and therapeutic services, support, information, advice and advocacy, as well as links to other sites, organisations and services.

- www.outsiders.org.uk/ Outsiders is another excellent website, founded by Dr Tuppy Owens. It works as an international social club for people with disability and also runs the Sex and Disability Helpline– a telephone-based support service staffed by both people with disabilities and health professionals.

- shada.org.uk The Sexual Health and Disability Alliance was instigated by Outsiders in 2005 to bring together those professionals who want to support the disabled people they work with in expressing themselves sexually.

Chapter 8
Way 40 Ageing and the Sexual Self

Online resources

The changes and health issues that many of us encounter as we age, such as joint pain, heart disease or surgery, don't have to mean an end to sex with our partners. For information for older people, their friends, family and carers about how to maintain an active, comfortable and safe sex life into old age, including advice on how to talk to partners about sex, Age UK is a good starting point: www.ageuk.org.uk/latest-press/archive/shhhhsex-doesnt-stop-in-your-60s is a valuable resource. The Age UK website also has a useful guide to dating in later life which covers internet dating, safety tips and same sex relationships: www.ageuk.org.uk/health-wellbeing/relationships-and-family/guide-to-dating

Not strictly speaking about sexuality but certainly about dispelling unhelpful myths around ageing, everybody, of any age, should watch the inspirational *Fabulous Fashionistas*, (www.channel4.com/programmes/fabulous-fashionistas), a Cutting Edge documentary shown by Channel 4 which introduces six stylish, inspirational women with an average age of 80, from different backgrounds and current circumstances.

Chapter 9
Way 42 Yoga and the sexual you

For more information on yoga see www.emmacoleyoga.com